A Child
Shall Lead Them

Books by Diane M. Komp, M.D.:

A Window to Heaven:
   When Children See Life in Death
A Child Shall Lead Them: Lessons in Hope
   from Children with Cancer

A Child Shall Lead Them

Lessons in Hope from Children with Cancer

DIANE M. KOMP, M.D.

ZondervanPublishingHouse
Grand Rapids, Michigan

HarperSanFrancisco
San Francisco, California

Divisions of HarperCollins*Publishers*

A Child Shall Lead Them:
Lessons in Hope from Children with Cancer
Copyright © 1993 by Diane M. Komp, M.D.
All rights reserved.

Co-published by Zondervan Publishing House
and HarperSanFrancisco.

Requests for information should be addressed to:
Zondervan Publishing House
Grand Rapids, Michigan 49530

Library of Congress Cataloging-in-Publication Data

Komp, Diane M.
    A child shall lead them : lessons in hope from children with cancer / Diane M.
Komp.
        p.   cm.
    ISBN 0-310-37980-6
    1. Tumors in children—Case studies. 2. Tumors in children—Religious
aspects—Christianity.   I. Title.
RC281.C4K62   1993
362.1'9892994–dc20   93–15642
                                                                              CIP

Edited by Lyn Cryderman
Interior design by Bob Hudson
Cover design by Jerry Fahselt
Cover illustration by Korene Mosher

93 94 95 96 97 98 /❖ BP / 7 6 5 4 3 2 1

For Katherine, Ryan, Sue,
and Barry

But if we hope for what we do not
see, we wait for it with patience.

Romans 8:24b–25 (NRSV)

Contents

Author's Preface

Several years ago, a former professor posed a challenge to me. "What do you collect?" he asked.

He, a world traveler, filled his home with priceless relics of many visits to the Far East. I don't collect objects of art, as he does. I collect stories. Stories about children are my treasure.

I told some of these stories in *A Window to Heaven*, a book that shared the spiritual experiences of youngsters facing death. This book is different. It draws from what children have taught me about living. You may notice a strong element of paradox winding through these tales. They reverse commonly held biases about illness, about life, about death. Perhaps you hold some of those biases as well.

Although names and minor events have been changed in many stories so that individual cases can remain anonymous, I have shared the narrative with the families involved wherever possible and appropriate. In a few cases a particular story is a composite.

In this book about hope, I deliberately included

the journeys of children who are still under treatment, stories whose final chapter remains unwritten. We need to learn how to live with uncertainty. Hope that is seen is not hope; this is a book about hope.

A major source of inspiration for this book comes from the growing numbers of long-term survivors of childhood cancer in my care. One mother refers to them as my "Olympic gold-medal winners." They are the unsung heroes and heroines of the cancer story. In a sense, this book is their song.

If you are looking for a counter-culture treatment of medicine and spirituality, you won't find it here. Most of my patients seek their health care within the mainstream of the "medical establishment," and their families ask their spiritual questions within the framework of the Judeo-Christian tradition. These are my matrices as well. I have chosen to write about their lives and mine from the point of view of a seasoned pediatrician and a faithful Christian. I encourage my readers to ask what it means for you to be seasoned and faithful.

Finally, I offer a list of those loyal friends and associates who also made this book possible. My pastors, Ken Norris and Peg Stearn, remain reliable sources of quotable quotes and loving support. Susan Lott Norris offered wise words about motherhood. There are no words that can adequately express my gratitude to Philip Yancey for being the special friend he is. Thanks are again due to Lyn Cryderman and Scott Bolinder at Zondervan for their continuing support and growing friendship and to my new partners at HarperSanFrancisco, Beth Webber and Tom Grady.

My deepest gratitude is to the children, their parents, and my colleagues at Yale. They share the work, the pain, the joy, and the hope. *They join in the song and help me to carry the tune.*

Diane M. Komp, New Haven, CT

Acknowledgments

Parts of this book were published in a series of essays in *Theology Today* entitled *A Mystery Story: Children, Cancer, and Covenant* , copyright 1989 by Diane M. Komp; *The Apple Doll House: Lessons from the Handicapped,* copyright 1990 by Diane M. Komp, and *Invitation to a Simple Feast,* copyright 1992 by Diane M. Komp. An article entitled, "Pediatric Cancer: Beating the Odds," was published in *Virginia Medical Monthly* 1979; 106:856–57, copyright 1979 by the Medical Society of Virginia. An essay entitled, "Lessons from Long-Term Survivors of Childhood Cancer" was published in *Pediatrics* 1989; 84, 910–11, copyright 1989 by the American Academy of Pediatrics.

Quotations from the Bible include *The New Revised Standard Version* (NRSV), copyright 1990 by the National Council of Churches of Christ in the United States of America; *The New International Version*® (NIV®), copyright 1973, 1978, 1984 by the International Bible Society; *The Jerusalem Bible* (JB), text, copyright 1966, 1967, and 1968 by Dartman, Longman & Todd, Ltd. and Doubleday & Co., Inc.

——— Prologue: ———

Let Me Tell You About My Grandchildren

*Blessed be childhood, which brings
down something of heaven into the
midst of our rough earthliness.*

Henri Frédéric Amiel

*D*ear Crumb-bunny,
   On the day of your bone marrow transplantation, I must tell you what a very special
baby you are. And very, very blessed. Sitting by your
crib, writing a letter in your Book of Hope, I imagine
that you will read these words on your wedding day.

   This disease that brought you to death's portal
(and to my office door) comes to only one in a million
babies. Most of them die. I am determined that you will
be a bride.

   You are special because, in a manner of speaking,
you have five living grandparents. When I was born,
only one of my grandparents was still alive. I will tell
you how your doctor got to be your extra grandma.
First, let me tell you a bedtime story, a tale of princesses
and of grandmas.

   A mommy asked her little girl what she wanted to
be when she grew up. The child thought for a while,
taking her time to answer, as little girls will. "I want to
be a princess," she said. "And a grandma."

"What does a princess do?" her mother inquired. Her daughter confidently replied, "A princess wears beautiful long dresses and dances all day in a wonderful castle!" Her eyes widened and she looked away, mistily and mysteriously dreaming of her future castle.

"And what does a grandmother do?" probed her mother. That took a bit more contemplation. "A grandma does the dishes and makes the beds and washes the windows ... Maybe I'll just be a princess!"[1] Let me tell you, Princess, this grandma doesn't wash windows! But grandmas have more in our job description than that little princess knew. Grandmothers are keepers of the family history and folklore. We like to link the past to the present while we rock little princesses in our ample bosoms.

To be a grandma is to be a storyteller. To be a princess is to be the story.

᠊᠊᠊   ᠊   ᠊

The headline on the early evening news was riveting: HISTORY IS BEING MADE TODAY AT YALE-NEW HAVEN HOSPITAL. We were gathered together in the Bone Marrow Transplantation Unit, savoring a moment of victory, watching a year of our collective lives unfold on television in sixty-second sound bites.

An anchorwoman titillated her viewers, warning that some of the scenes to follow would be "graphic." File footage of an operating room filled the screen with the image of a patient anesthetized upon a table, sterilely draped, poised for action. Steel needles flashed, glass syringes shimmered, dramatic tension peaked. Attention focused on the sleeping bone-marrow donor, a gifter of life.

"So that's how it's done!" observed a bald man on the other side of a plastic barrier from us. "I've never seen how they actually get the bone marrow." Medical staff and family of a mortally ill baby whom I had nicknamed Crumb-bunny, huddled outside a yellow line to watch the news.

It was, in fact, a patient billeted inside the protective environment of a Bone Marrow Transplant room who was speaking to us. We were his guests-at-a-safe-distance for the early evening news. A yellow line, the border of no-man's-land, separated us from this young businessman in his "life island." Were we to step over the line, his life would be in danger.

As the story unrolled, this young man himself appeared on the TV screen, the camera skillfully shooting through the protective, transparent partition. The news team had interviewed him earlier in the day and learned his own happy story. He was close to discharge time now, his brother's donated cells willingly repopulating his own empty marrow space.

A few doors away, another story was just beginning. A baby played in her crib. She, a newcomer to this alien world, had a long road ahead. We don't often have such very young children in the Bone Marrow Unit. The staff had lovingly decorated the baby's cubicle with all the care that first-time parents devote to their firstborn child's nursery. Sterile need not translate as impersonal.

But we were not the only players in this prime-time drama. Barely 200 miles away, a helicopter was meeting a British jumbo jet at Kennedy Airport, delivering our nurse Hanne and a priceless gift-harvest for the seventeen-month-old infant. Hanne hadn't bargained for a helicopter ride when she accepted the assignment to hand-carry the life-saving gift all the way from a British operating theater. We all wanted to see the blush on her cheeks when she finally landed and saw all the TV cameras and all of us.

We had waited an entire year for this day. The baby was born healthy but became sick shortly thereafter. Three years earlier, her brother died soon after birth from the same strange illness. It was not until she came to us that the correct diagnosis, a one-in-a-million genetic disease, was suspected.

For many years my research has focused on a peculiar and rare disease known as "histiocytosis."[2] The baby had the most rare and deadly form of this disease. Until the last few years, all babies born with this form of histiocytosis, like her brother, eventually died. But now there was hope.

It was exhilarating to read the early reports in medical journals of a possible cure. Bone marrow transplantation—taking cells from a healthy brother or sister and giving it to the sick child—was a relatively new way to manage this disease. This baby had no surviving sibling, no such match. And this awful disease, held in check by chemotherapy, was starting to come back.

Sadly, we were aware of many infants who died before finding unrelated donors. Turning from the small, intimate family circle to a vast uncaring world is an act of desperate hope. Would a stranger care enough about a stranger? Could we find a donor in time?

There was cause for celebration that evening. There was just such a caring person, thousands of miles away. A perfectly matched but unrelated bone marrow donor had been located in England, renewing hope for our baby.

Now it was time to mobilize. As we waited for the bone marrow to arrive, the staff of *Guideposts* magazine gathered in their corporate offices to pray for her. Members of the family's church organized an all-day prayer vigil. Days before, we had treated the baby with lethal doses of chemotherapy, making room in her small body for the new bone marrow.

As she waved at me through the plastic curtain, it was hard to grasp how absolutely defenseless she was against common germs in ordinary air, clear tap water. The whir of a laminar air-flow fan was a sinister reminder of her total vulnerability.

At six o'clock we all rushed out to the hospital helipad together, waving and giggling and hugging each other like happy fools, shading our eyes from the sunset. The journalists beat us and had cameras and notebooks poised for the dramatic moment when our nurse would emerge from the chopper.

Lenses zoomed in on the delivery to Dr. Joel Rappeport, then swept to the young parents. They told of searching the world for a suitable donor for their only surviving child. Mom and Dad said they believed that this moment was an answer to prayer.

One of the media herd noticed my enthusiastic enjoyment of the moment and hoped there might be another story here to the side of the crowd. "Who are you?" she asked, "The baby's grandmother?"

My colleagues stared at her in disbelief. When she heard my name and realized who I was, she stammered an apology and mumbled her congratulations to the entire medical team.

Later that evening, my car crossed the Quinnipiac Bridge that spans my two worlds. On this twilight re-entry from high-tech hospital to hemlock-guarded hideaway, I thought about her words. Surely there must have been something in my expression that led her to conclude that I was the baby's grandmother.

What a superb compliment it was, this suspicion of grandmotherliness. And what a rare opportunity it now provides. Years ago I began talking of the off-spring of my long-term surviving patients as my "grandchildren." Now that I'm getting older, even my patients' parents are young enough to be my children. If you have a few hours, dear reader, let me tell you about these grandchildren. Let me share my world with you.

Set your presumptions aside about sickness and death, children and cancer. Prepare yourself for paradox. Where you suppose death to rule, life abounds. Where you expect pathos, there may be humor in its place. Children will lead and wise adults will follow. Leave your biases at the door. And take off your shoes, for this is holy ground. But you are safe and welcome. It is only your presumptions you need to leave behind.

1

A Child Shall Lead Them

A door had opened in the universe, and through my son, and in my face. The Glory of the Lord had burst from a little child.

Walter Wangerin, Jr.

*D*ear Crumb-bunny,
 Precious, irreplaceable, vulnerable and mortally ill you were when we first met. I adored you at first sight, made you part of our family. I brooded over the grim medical facts of your case and watched my colleagues mentally hang a crêpe over your crib.

 Because of your diagnosis, my co-workers saw you as good as dead. Statistically, they were entitled to that opinion. But I aimed to transpose gloom into hope, hope into action. This was the genesis of your Book of Hope.

 Today, your day of hope, is a time to say "thank you." First, let me thank you for coming into my life, enriching it. But I am not your only admirer. Taped near your crib is a card from your donor with her blessings for you. She signed her first name, and we have formed mental pictures of this woman we have come to love like a sister. Your parents have organized a package of thank-you notes to send her. The British bone-marrow registry will forward our thanks to her. Thus far there are more than 100 cards to send.

Babies can make adults do the most unusual things that we just won't do for each other. As long as there are babies, there will be hope.

> ❧　　❧　　❧

I didn't start my medical studies intending to be a pediatrician of any sort, much less a specialist in children's cancer.[3] Yet, at 3:00 A.M. in December last year, I found myself in a hospital emergency room, preparing to inflict pain on a stranger's child.

"Matt, I have to give you a shot," I prepared him as I ripped open an alcohol wipe. The medicinal sting in my nose revived a long-forgotten memory. When I was Matt's age, my own pediatrician planned to give me a simple shot of penicillin. To attempt this, he had to chase me around an examining table. The old sport wasn't up to the chase the day of my reckoning and quit after a few sweaty laps. Frustrated and irritated, he suspended further efforts to corral me. He informed my mother that my hysteria would neutralize the antibiotic even if he gave it. My adrenaline, he alleged, could undo the wonder drug's wonder. Even then I could spot a pharmacological fib.

Matt gave me a merry chase in the months to follow his rite of passage on that bleak midwinter night. He reminded me what it is like to be a frightened child. I recall his father's love and his mother's determination. His mother will not let me give up on the chase, and I will not fib.

His mother stayed with him for all painful procedures we performed to save Matt's life. When I looked up from my instruments, I could see her practicing her tigress look. When you're a mother, you sometimes have to think with your claws. When I finished, I saw the tears form in her eyes as she whispered "thank you."

I never considered making my baby doctor's career my own. In medical school a professor of pediatrics reinforced this disinclination. During my apprenticeship on a children's ward, I sat at a nurses' station listening to his unsolicited advice.

"Don't go into pediatrics," he advised, punctuating his professorial counsel with a paternal pat on my hand. "Women shouldn't be exposed to suffering children." He was serious. He meant to persuade.

Assurances followed. He pointed to his own daughter, a doctor. He saw himself as an authentic believer, not an arrant bigot. He saw a place for women in medicine but not in pediatrics.

He had steered his daughter (and hoped to lead me) away from his own special field. Mysteries were safer with men, I imagined him to imagine. Rachel might weep for her children because they are no more.

Suffering and death can be deep, deep mysteries indeed. As a student, my greatest fear was that I might weep. I imagined that the faculty watched the rare women students, waiting for the waterworks to begin, and I did not want to give them ammunition for their biases.

An instructor in pharmacology was distraught when I wept over a dog used for a laboratory experiment. The instructor said that they had never taught him in graduate school what to do about such situations. I took that to mean that he didn't know what to do about women students. Tears and chaos that had erupted in his lab.

I caught the expression on his face and never wept again. I thought of that day as I listened to my newest instructor. Was this pediatrician a prophet, anticipating the dark night of the soul ahead for me? Or was he simply a kinder and gentler sexist?

The scene at the nurses' station so long ago was one of those magic moments of mentoring, how young doctors learn the art of medicine. We learn by the example of others, what they choose to share. Thirty years later, at a different nurses' station in another hospital, I am the baby doctor, the professor, the mentor. I face a suffering boy who must suffer more before daylight comes. A young medical student sits near me, observing my every move.

My earnest dissuader in medical school was the first but not my only instructor in the health care of children. In that mammoth city hospital, young pediatricians-in-training tried to persuade me to join their happy ranks. The pediatric residents were happy zealots, looking for new comrades.

Pediatrics was one of the few departments in that teaching hospital without a jail ward. In that sprawling haven for the suffering poor, there never were enough beds for all those in need. Prison bars may have been missing from the outer perimeters of the pediatric wards, but the lives of many of the little ones were similarly governed by circumstances over which they had no control.

Trapped by poverty, the parents seemed as powerless as their babes. In this department where you learned how to change a diaper before you learned how to change medication orders, I met senior doctors who were convinced that they could make a difference in a sad, sad world. And the most outrageous Don Quixote of them all was in charge.

The chief pediatrician had high expectations from us. He assumed that we knew all the scientific minutiae. He was more interested to hear what we had learned as human beings. He wasn't content to let invisible bars confine him and the babes in his charge. Once he had even taken on City Hall on behalf of youngsters whose bones and brains were filled with an urban poison. Lead poisoning could be today's death or tomorrow's learning disability, but this doctor simply would not let the children go home to die by either route.

As medical students, we could recite all the biochemical esoterica, the enzymatic blocks by which the damage is done. But if we had no comprehension of the social implications of the illness—of how lead actually got into the systems of these children—we had failed in his view.

The pediatric bed-census validated his claims.

Our wards were always full of these children, long after they were well enough for discharge. Tenement housing, the source of their ailments, had low priority with the bureaucrats. One month before I started pediatrics, I completed an assignment in community health, visiting a family who lived in this sort of subsidized squalor. The building was so dangerous that we sometimes borrowed a friend's German shepherd to make our house calls. Today, you would need an armed police escort.

I have seen firsthand the chips of old lead-based paint that peel off the walls and find their way into hungry mouths, growing brains. No one listened to the impoverished tenants when they complained. They were welfare clients, after all. Their caseworkers reminded them of how fortunate they were to even have roof over their heads.

A "hot line" linked Dr. Lanman's office to the Health Department laboratory where they tested blood lead levels. He refused to discharge a child from our hospital until the housing was safe. Since the city could not afford for our acute beds to be filled with chronic cases, an inspector was promptly dispatched to the home to facilitate repairs. This good doctor used his power to assist the powerless and won.

My hero was a dashing silver fox in long, white cotton twill. We murmured to each other as he strode down the hall, recounting tales of all the windmills he had successfully slain. I was the chief murmurer.

On the pediatric wards I felt free to be myself. My infatuation with a baby hospitalized for heart problems was no great secret. Her mother was so afraid that Milagros would die that she never visited her child. When the nurses called me about her medical care, they would refer to me as her "mother."

My own income was below poverty level that year, but I bought a secondhand sewing machine and made elegant lace-trimmed nightgowns for my lovely new Hispanic "daughter." I was always partial to lace, and so was Milly. She was very proud and pranced in her crib, fussing with the lace.

I always assumed that my extra-curricular stitches were my secret, known only to the nurses. My assumption proved flawed when the senior doctors joined us one day for rounds. As we came to Milly's crib, I stood to the rear of the group lest the baby and the nurses betray me.

The chief unbuttoned the lace ribbon at her neckline to listen to her heart. Then he turned to find me. "Dr. Komp, I recognize your suturing when I see it. I assume that you will be carrying this baby along with us for the rest of our rounds. The next time, just get her before we start. Milly shouldn't have to wait so long for her 'mother' to collect her."

This regal gentleman did not pat hands. If he was a father figure, he was the sort who blessed and released. He blessed me by his example and released me to chart my own way. Yet I still had no serious thoughts about pediatrics for a career.

❧   ❧   ❧

Never did I hear a word of direct advice from my next teacher, the person whose opinion meant the most to me. For four happy weeks I worked with an eminent physician who had escaped from an oppressive regime to start his professional life over in America.

Although trained as an internist, Ramon Torres became a heart specialist for children and found himself most at home with youngsters and their advocates. To complete his American credentials, he had to step away from a senior faculty position for a year and become a resident. When I was a student, he was my supervising pediatric resident. I followed him everywhere, and he simply taught me everything that he knew about children.

Would I choose internal medicine or pediatrics? I agonized over my career decision until the deadline for internship applications. The younger residents tried to coax; Torres never said a word.

I cannot remember the exact sequence of thoughts that led to the most important career decision I've ever made. It seemed as if the heavens had opened and a big sign with the word PEDIATRICS emblazoned upon it was lowered for my viewing. I ran to Dr. Torres' office with the revelation.

"Diane, Diane!" he laughed, shaking his head.

"You were the only one who didn't know you were going into pediatrics." That day I completed my applications for a pediatric residency, a decision I've never regretted.

és   és   és

Now, at 3:00 A.M., I am in another hospital with a different pediatric resident at my side. He is weary from long hours, worried about Matt, and very alarmed at the diagnosis I suspect. The yellow cast to the child's skin, the balloon-tight belly, his pain-haunted eyes—they all spell malignancy. Not school phobia as the first doctor suspected, nor hepatitis as the second one had hoped.

This young resident chose pediatrics because he supposed that children only get quick-fix illnesses, if they get sick at all. Sneeze one day, play the next. Cancer is an obscenity that should happen to no one, much less a child. Neither should a stranger inflict more pain on a little stranger. Nor should parents need to scrutinize a doctor's eyes in search of truth and hope. I know his thoughts (they once were mine).

Our job together, learner and mentor, is to fight for Matt's life. In striving together all night this night, hopefully I will pass on something worth learning. And I will not pat his hand.

és   és   és

My career "revelation" solved one dilemma but it left another in its place. The mystery of suffering continued to loom, unresolved, threatening. Because of my own choice, no one could protect me from little ones who suffer. But I still demanded an answer about their suffering. Both science and religion had led me to believe that questions had answers. My quest led past the children and their parents—to God. And there the buck stopped . . . with God.

Beholding the mystery, my faith began to flounder. A boy with hemophilia injured himself every Christmas to come to our hospital. Our "home" was happier than his. Leukemia filled a little girl's brain, leaving her with hallucinations about horrible bugs crawling on her skin. We gave her a tranquilizer. The imaginary bugs remained, but she no longer cared about them. Where was the hope for these children?

Surely, lambs and lions could not lie together, as some silly prophet had once declared![4] From my vantage point, God seemed to be flogging the lambs instead of the lions. How could a rational person believe in such a deity? How shall I find my own way in this jungle, much less lead little lambs to safety?

What lay ahead in the jungle for me was to learn that it was not I who would lead the children home. *It would be the children who would lead me instead.*

— 2 —

Let My Heart
Be Broken

*The heart must break or become
as bronze.*

Chamfort

*D*ear Crumb-bunny,
  I asked all your doctors and nurses to write notes in your Book of Hope for you to read when you grow up. To envision you grown up—Crumb-bunny in a bridal gown rather than a burial shroud—takes a leap of faith. In recent years, faith has not been a notable component of medical tradition.

As they struggled to find the words for your Book of Hope, I watched the attitude on the ward miraculously start to change. I saw a subtle, even a hopeful progression in the notes they entered in your medical chart as well. Doctors and nurses joined us in the sweet conspiracy, the daring hope, the outrageous consideration that you might survive. They did not want their hearts to be broken.

When I was little, they used to say about a particularly sweet girl-child that when she grew up she would break men's hearts. You, little flirt, have those kinds of looks. But of you they say, "If she doesn't grow up, it will break my heart."

There are many adults I know who try to shield themselves from such heartbreak. Your mother, dear child, is not one of them. For a child, her own or someone else's, she will always take a risk.

There's a sweetness to your mom that I hope you have inherited. As sick as you are and as sad as your own family's story has been, she has always cared about all the children who come to our clinic. Your mother's attitude reminds me of a saying I heard many years ago: "Let my heart be broken with the thing that breaks the heart of God."[5]

ૐ ૐ ૐ

Perhaps my first pediatric teacher was right. To be exposed to suffering children is a dangerous proposition. As children died, my faith seemed to be perish as well. To handle the pain, I took the advice of a professor of internal medicine.

He was doing his best to counsel young students as he rounded with us on our patients. He advised us not to heed the pain that our feelings bring when we listen to our patients. We should simply do our work and concentrate on that. Hard work is a good tonic for untamed and uneasy feelings. There was plenty of work, ample opportunity to concentrate away from the untidy arena of emotion.

Yet there's a critical distinction between suspending feelings for the moment and denying that they ever held any import. This professor never tried to make such a distinction, but I believe he shared as best he knew. Feelings were the purview of social workers, not doctors, he thought.

Empathy, what most patients long for from their doctors, is defined as "the identification with, and understanding of another's situation, *feelings*, and motives."[6] For me, the denial of full-bodied empathy to my patients was a personal loss as well. It spelled the difference between spiritual life and death.

True empathy resonates with life's most profound questions. *It is only when we share the feelings of another that we understand the importance of hope. Without hope, we cannot live. Without hope, we are already dead.* Of course, we could choose work that keeps us away from dying patients altogether. Where is it written, thou shalt be a masochist?

I learned to work unflogged by untidy feelings. But everytime I considered taking a "safe" course, to avoid the suffering of children, the path led away from the most joyous parts of medicine as well. There were mysteries within the mystery.

ð≥ ð≥ ð≥

There was a particular boy with leukemia I met when I was an intern who seemed destined to die. *If he must die,* I thought, *let it be peaceful.* An oncologist came along with a drug so new that it was still considered investigational. Vincristine was unlikely to cure his disease, but it was certain to make his hair fall out.

I wondered about this peculiar breed of pediatricians who gave "poisons" to mere babes. We students and residents gossiped about these ghouls behind their backs, yet they seemed to be the only members of the faculty that we saw after midnight. Their patients and the parents received them as members of the family, even seemed to love them. They seemed to bring hope with their words and their protocols. *There must be something about their job,* I thought, *that we fledgling baby-docs did not yet understand.*

It was this speciality that attracted me most, even though it threatened the most exposure to suffering in children. Remember, this was a quarter century ago, when few children with cancer survived these treatments. It defies logic why I made the choice.

I entered the field with the intention to pursue laboratory-based work, safe from baldness and tears. I also reasoned that this would be the likeliest place to find a solution to the puzzle of disease. This was the sort of hope a scientist could understand. In my childhood, science had saved children from polio. Now science could address the next important plague: cancer.

But science failed regularly. I risked drowning in a sea of malignant ifs. If I was smarter. If I had read just one more article. If I had stayed up a few more hours. Rather than drown, I swam back to the safety of the lab. When I did work with the kids, I did my best, secure in the knowledge that I could keep my safe distance. Someone else was ultimately responsible.

As a junior faculty member, I was able to maintain this distance until an unexpected turn of events. The colleague who did most of the clinical work in our department left for another medical school. But his patients stayed behind.

At first I made plans to recruit another doctor to take care of the clinical work. To my amazement, I found that the closer I got to children with cancer, the easier the job was. Instead of sapping my energy, these kids were life-giving. The malignant ifs were transmutated into peace of mind. Gladly, the job close to the children became mine.

Ș Ș Ș

Instead of expecting a miracle worker, the children with cancer and their parents seemed satisfied with a fellow sojourner. If I did my best, that sufficed. What was important to them was that we were there together. One young mother and her firstborn son made a profound impression on me. So vivid is my memory of her that I used her for the prototype for Sarah in *Facing Mount Moriah*,[7] a chapter in my previous book.

It was this young family who motivated me to support home care for dying children long before we in America heard about hospice. It was children like her own who showed me a window to heaven, full of hope, dreams, visions, and faith.

From this young mother I learned that there are wiser teachers than the professors. You can recognize them by the diaper bags they carry. Near the time of her son's death, she spoke of another young doctor who suffered because of her own sense of inadequacy. "I wanted to tell her that she would be okay—there would be another patient for her to care for. But of course, at the time I couldn't find the words to say it." *My professors were not half as wise as she.*

Today more than half of young people diagnosed with cancer will survive without any evidence of disease recurrence. The news is especially good for children with some forms of leukemia where the expectations are that 80% of them will live to tell the story about their victories. There is even better news about infants with a common form of malignant tumor when limited to the kidney. For them, the cure rate approaches 100%. Every year the report gets better. Even for Matt.

Matt went directly from Emergency to our Intensive Care Unit. My worst fear was realized when the biopsy came back as Burkitt's lymphoma. This malignancy grows so fast that some of these children die in the first few days. The first early days were not very pleasant, but Matt's parents were there at his side. That made all the unpleasantries do-able.

It takes many different doctors and a team of nurses to pull such a child through. When the chemo started to work, Matt's health and smile returned simultaneously. He has a wonderful, nine-year-old boy's smile, auguring mischief as well as remission. Six months later, his treatment is complete. No Burkitt's cells can be found.

Matt celebrates his latest good report by joining a panel of adult cancer survivors, telling participants in an international congress that they can ask him any questions they desire. There's no question too painful if he might help someone else. He is happy to be there; his parents beam with pride. On my twenty-fifth anniversary as a pediatric oncologist, I am proud as well.

ðŸ€   ðŸ€   ðŸ€

The good news does not stop with the improvements in treatment. Supported by the company of the children, I started to ask questions again of God. I heard no voice from heaven, but I did hear the voice of the children. It was through their voices that I understood what Jesus meant when he said, "And remember, I am with you always, to the end of the age."[8] *These are words full of hope.*

I have never regretted the choice of oncology for a career. It's been my privilege to participate in three of the fastest-moving decades in cancer treatment and make my own small contributions to the progress. It is not professional success that keeps me in the field. It is the children.

Tonight I think back on the pain that I tried to avoid by distancing myself from these children and realize how much greater the pain of avoidance is than that of their embrace. I hear the echo of my own once-breaking heart in a voice on my telephone answering-machine.

It was hard to hear the entire message because of the choked-back tears that punctuated his words. The caller was a middle-aged man who identified himself as a pastor in the Midwest. He was distraught. A little child in his congregation had an aggressive tumor, and nothing in seminary or three decades of parish ministry had prepared him for this painful experience. He had never dealt with a child with cancer before.[9]

As we spoke, he stammered with emotion but managed to tell me about the child's family. Their community doctor had sent them to a major pediatric cancer center. The staff of the big center were marvelous and supportive, he said. The parents were doing fine. He referred to them as "bearers of the holy." But the pastor's heart was breaking. A member of his church was suffering, and he felt impotent. He seemed to be suffering more than the sufferer.

A pastor weeps. Yet parents rise up with wings as eagles. Young doctors with other options count themselves privileged to cast their lot with these children. And middle-aged physicians like me can find our way back to faith when we listen to such children.

Therein is the paradox: *The closer you come to these children, the less the pain. If you risk letting your heart be broken, you just may find it healed.*

3

Isaac's Return from Mount Moriah

This strange tale is about fear and faith, fear and defiance, fear and laughter. Terrifying in content, it has become a source of consolation to those who, in retelling it, make it part of their own experience.

Elie Wiesel

*D*ear Crumb-bunny,
  Unlike a medical chart, your Book of Hope is beautiful enough for a bride. This floral-fabric journal is your hospital guest-book for visitors. The book was my idea, but it was your mother's notion to bring hope into its title. My billets-doux are a different type of medical progress note.

  Your story, little one, reminds me of a biblical one, of Abraham and Isaac on the path up to Mount Moriah. As the story goes, God asked a man of faith to sacrifice his only living son. St. Paul said that Abraham hoped against hope that Isaac would survive.

  You may have noticed that your parents are people of faith. But would they take you and risk your life if they did not trust God? For most parents, the analogy of Mount Moriah is an incomplete one. Few parents I meet as a doctor get to exercise free choice. Most just find themselves there on the mountain, forced to decide under pressure. Your own Abraham and Sarah know the metaphor in full.

  As long as you were sick, the decision to accept the

chemotherapy was an easy one. There was no other choice for sane parents. They made a date to deliver you up, signed consent for the lethal doses of even more powerful drugs to be administered to wipe out your own bone marrow. This is strong stuff for doctors, let alone parents.

The medications to destroy your own bone marrow began days before Nurse Hanne winged her way over to London. What if the donor had second thoughts and backed out? What if Hanne tripped and dropped the container with the marrow?

Mommy and Daddy hope against hope. They are at peace with God's loving care for you.

ê&   ê&.   ê&

In *A Window to Heaven* I compared the plight of such parents to the situation of Abraham and Sarah and Isaac on Mount Moriah. The majority of the children I described in that book did not return from the Mount. This book has a different emphasis, so my metaphoric Isaac shall return.

A few small rocks are the first to break the silence, and then an unmodulated voice of a young lad is heard as he races down the hillside. Sarah's voice echoes as she calls after him, "Isaac! Don't run so fast. You haven't even walked for a month. Isaac! Where are you?"

His face is flushed with excitement as he races up to me. "Dr. Di, did you see what happened on the mountain? Awesome! Hey, I'm hungry. I could eat a whole cow. You got any peanut butter crackers? Awesome!"

Sarah and Abraham reach the foot of the mountain, nod to me briefly, and then head for home. There are no words that need to be said. Their Isaac is safe.

Snug in his bed, surrounded by a legion of stuffed animals, Isaac snores softly. Sarah sits on the edge of the bed running her fingers through his curly hair. It had been straight before the treatment, but now there are these handsome curls.

The first stage is what we call the "chemo cut." In the summer, the chemo cut bleaches out on the tips. It's hard to overcome the temptation to run your fingers through the thick pelt that eventually replaces the bald pate.

Little boys roll their eyes when mothers and doctors give in to the tactile temptation. In this sense we love being weak. As the child sleeps soundly, Sarah's resolve that never was dissolves. Her fingers plow rows through the dense rich crown. They are a symbol of hope.

Abraham joins her at his side and they watch Isaac sigh. In his sleep, he clutches the teddy bear he got after his last bone marrow. One for every marrow, another for each spinal, Isaac sleeps in a zoological garden. When he goes off to college, Sarah will take teddy and the others to her own room before her son discards them in a fit of pubertal machismo.

In the marital bed, Abraham and Sarah embrace each other tightly to shut out all that is not them and theirs and allow their eyes to fill to overflowing. Tears of relief, streams of repressed anger, rivers of joy flow that they have returned from Moriah with their family intact. Then their embrace broadens and with it their prayers for other families. Mostly they pray for Isaac, that he will always know how special he is to God. Then they sleep.

Sarah and Abraham will never forget where they have been, nor what has happened. Chances are that Isaac's memory will fade as he grows up.

Woody, a lively child, was just short of his third birthday when he developed leukemia and came into my care. Without coaching, he tuned out the pain from bone marrows and spinal taps. I gloved, and he snored. It was that simple. He never felt a thing.

When he was a mature man of five, he forgot all that and couldn't understand what we were talking about when we tried to remind him. Our social worker thought that nursery rhymes might be a suitable trick to help him regain what he had lost. An indignant pre-schooler listened suspiciously, then sputtered out, "I don't want no rock. I want Mozart!" For the next two years, I did his bone marrows to *Eine Kleine Nacht-musik*. Again, he never felt a thing.

Time passed and he became an old gent of twelve. When I told him that he needed a bone marrow, he howled and haggled. He shook his head at me once more, "You keep telling me about putting myself to sleep and doing bone marrows to Mozart. I don't remember that at all." His parents and I will always remember and wish he did, too.

In the land that gave us Sigmund Freud, I shared this story with pediatricians. The members of the Austrian Pediatric Society were less impressed with the point I intended to make about pain control than the musical message. In America there dwells one small child who prefers Mozart to rock!

I've known Woody for most of his life. He is proud that he is no longer a little boy. I've seen him grow into new skills but I've also seen him outgrow some of his earliest abilities. Woody has reached an age when he needs to be retaught some things that he once seemed to know intuitively. I wonder what or Whom he knew that helped him so much when he was so young.

I heard a story recently about a three-year-old who wanted to spend time with his new baby brother. "I want to be alone with the baby," he insisted. We can only wonder what concerns of sibling rivalry raced through his parents' minds as they listened to this modest but pregnant request.

The child was so earnest that they allowed him to remain alone in the room with the sleeping baby. With a sense of awe, he gently touched the sleeping baby and then begged quietly, "You've got to tell me about God. I'm beginning to forget already."[10]

Parents or religious instructors are not their true teachers. This holy imagination, a sense of spiritual origins, is intuitive in the very young. It is as if a veil descends thereafter, leaving the pilgrim in search of ways to reconnect. We older pilgrims must seek others who know the Story to tell us, too, if we would learn to hope.

Sometimes, as death approaches, the veil seems to lift in part, giving hints of that beyond, visions of angels, of Jesus, of heaven. Most of us are pilgrims in between, living with a sense of déjà vu, groping our way back to God.

≈ ≈ ≈

In her book, *Chasing the Dragon,* Jackie Pullinger tells a remarkable story about a four-year-old Chinese boy who was pronounced dead after a drowning accident.[11]

Later, he woke and told his mother of a man who had held out his hand and pulled him out of the water. His mother asked him if he knew the man's name, assuming that it was the headmaster of the school where the accident had occurred. "Don't you know?" replied the boy. "It's Jesus."

This family had fled from mainland China to Taiwan and never had contact with Christians. His mother, who had never before heard the name of Jesus, became a Christian as a result of this child's experience.

What is most remarkable about this story is the further history of the little boy.

Although his mother became a Christian, the boy himself went on to become a drug dealer. It was in a Hong Kong prison that Miss Pullinger met him. Despite his early "inspiring" experience, he himself had to reach rock bottom as an adult before his own life was changed spiritually.

Children who survive near-fatal illnesses are no more guaranteed than the rest of us to retain God-consciousness. Isaac returns from Moriah a healthier lad, but he, too, must choose to become faithful. Isaac must become a consenting adult to the life of faith himself for the covenant to be carried forward.

4

Beating the Odds

*My doctor's favorite plant is
the hedge.*

A child with cancer,
quoted by Erma Bombeck

*D*ear Crumb-bunny,
     *You peek through the layers of plastic that
     separate us until you can find me. Then you
smile and give one of your backward waves, admiring
your own fingers, the way you always wave. There
must be an interesting secret engraved on the palm of
your hand that you don't yet choose to share. Will you
ever wave the way that other babies do?*

*I am not a betting person and Sweetie, let me tell
you something else. Jimmie the Greek and most doctors
won't be betting on you this month. You are what they
call a "long shot."*

*Hope doesn't like to be estimated. It prefers to be
nonquantitatively enjoyed. The TV journalists pressed
Dr. Joel into making an on-camera guess at your odds.
Reluctantly, he said "50/50." We have a choice in how
we interpret these odds. We can either see the glass as
half empty or half full.*

*A year ago your chances were closer to zero, but
here you are. Now you know why I hedge. I don't like
statistics. You are a princess, not a race horse. When Joel*

looks at you, he gives you a 100% look. He seems to be by you 100% of his time these days.

What do you want to be when you grow up besides a princess and a grandma? I always think about your surviving, entitled to your dreams. Despite the deadly nature of your illness, I have always seen you as a living person. You are someone just like me; we are not different. One day you shall die; one day I shall die. Even there, we do not differ.

So, my love, what do you want to be when you grow up? Most of my patients imagine becoming doctors, play with stethoscopes as toys, and beg us for the biggest syringes we can find. They make the best squirt guns. Their dolls all have Hickman catheters under their dresses or IVs taped on their arms. You watch us and turn our medical mysteries into your play.

I think you'll do a better job than most of us when you take our place. You certainly have the heart for people. What do you carry away from us about life and death? What can you children offer your doctors to heal our own fear of death?

෫෧   ෫෧   ෫෧

When I was in medical school, few children with cancer survived and "cure" was not a word we used in the discussion of leukemia. I learned early not to play the numbers game.

As a resident, I dreaded the admission of a child with cancer to my ward and worried over what to say.

Even as a young faculty member, I avoided statistics in discussing prognosis. Until recently, Crumb-bunny's disease was 100% fatal and in many hospitals it still is.

Today in my office I have the privilege to see many young people who had cancer but are now what we call "long-term survivors." They have completed their treatment and are going on with their lives. When many of them first were ill, the percentages didn't promise much. But here they are today, 100% here. I offer them annual appointments until they want to "fire" me for an internist. Most of them stay on unless they move out of the area.

Recently, there was close to a convention of long-term survivors at my clinic. I had a bumper-crop of college freshmen this year, the sort who passionately celebrate life. These kids easily mix with the younger new ones, playing the big brother or sister. *They are a living memorial to the power of hope.*

The chemo room that they once dreaded no longer holds power over them—they are not the ones hooked up to tubing. But it was in just such a room that they became survivors. If they can help someone else who is just starting in, they will. For the sake of another, their old fear is canceled and they cross the threshold that once brought a bilious taste to their mouths.

When I left my previous academic post to come to Yale, I entitled my last "grand rounds" there, "Pediatric Cancer: Beating the Odds"[12] Three of my long-term survivors participated in that teaching conference. By odds, none of them should be alive. There was something particularly mean about each of their tumors that said at the outset that the odds were against them. All of these kids had outlived cancer and were off therapy for several years at the time they shared the podium with me.

A decade later I was reminded of that particular grand rounds by a telephone call on my birthday. Although I hadn't seen him for ten years, his voice was unmistakable. How can you forget the voice of the first leukemia patient you were able to tell that he was cured? Freddie was also the first of my long-term survivors to become a parent and supply me with "grandchildren" to brag about.

Freddie started with leukemia as a teenager. He is now forty years old and a coal miner. In the town where he lived, only the mines provided health benefits for someone with a history of malignancy. Freddie was realistic and in love. He didn't want to jeopardize his young family.

When Freddie was first sick, his father tried to withhold the truth from him and even denied to him that he had leukemia. The son rebelled by not taking all his prescribed medications. When he confided this to me many years later, he told me that he knew that his father meant well. But his dad had not handled the situation in a way that was in his best interests.

I thought that this was an important message, one worth sharing with other parents who face the same situation that his father faced. I arranged to videotape an interview with Freddie. As things worked out, this did not take place until the death of his father and the birth of his first child. I have never been able to use the video for its intended purpose.

On-camera I heard that parents always know what is best for their children; parents are always right. Teenagers don't know what they're talking about; they should be obedient and grateful. Now that Freddie's own children are teenagers, I wonder what he was experiencing that day of my birthday that lead him to reach out by telephone to someone who was important to him when he was the age of his children?

His children, my first "grandchildren," are already teenagers and there have been dozens more born since then to other patients. More than one is named Diane. I pulled out the details of those old grand rounds on my birthday, enjoying the excuse to reminisce.

Harold was only three years old when he had Hodgkin's disease. Thereafter, it recurred many times to treatment. His parents agreed to try a brand-new medication as part of a research trial. This research drug had much the same status that vincristine had when I was an intern—unproven, not all side effects yet known. There was nothing else we could offer. This time I was the "ghoul," and new interns wondered if I had lost all common sense.

Harold not only achieved permanent remission, he has been disease-free now for twenty years. The medication he received, a new drug from Italy called adriamycin, proved to be one of the most important drugs in the history of chemotherapy. We had no way to know that then. We could only hope. Harold's mother called me a few years ago, simply to say, "I love you."

John was three when he developed lung metastases from a kidney tumor. He was already receiving the best chemotherapy we knew. I find it ironic as I reread the opening section of my grand rounds:

I want you to picture yourself as a parent. Your beautiful three-year-old daughter has not been her usual self. She appears tired and sallow to you, so you take her to your physician . . . . After an anxious wait, the verdict comes in from the laboratory. Your physician explains to you that this disease from which she suffers has no cure—but there are medications available to which 90-100% of similarly afflicted children respond. Once the disease remits, however, it will be necessary to continue medication or the disease will relapse.

The medication is not without side effects. The chances are now better than ever, you are told, that your daughter will live to adulthood. If she becomes pregnant, however, her pregnancies will be considered high risk; fetal wastage is a strong possibility, and birth defects have been reported in a significant number of offspring of mothers who have been similarly treated.

You, as a parent, ask what will happen if no treat-
ment is given. Spontaneous remissions are rare, you are
told, and without treatment, your daughter most cer-
tainly will die. What is your choice? How would you
weigh the preview of the quality of your child's life?
Why not allow her to slip away now rather than risk
toxic treatment of an "incurable" disease with potential
for death at a later point?

The radiologist who read John's chest film glared
at me as he looked at the white shadow on a black
background. There was no doubt that it was tumor. He
assumed that I would send him home to die and was
shocked to hear my plans.

"What do you mean, you're going to give more
chemotherapy and radiotherapy? He's only three years
old and he has no hope." John completed treatment
twenty years ago. He plans to apply to medical school
and his mother threatens to send him to live with me to
cut down on expenses.

The rest of the introduction to that grand rounds
extends the irony by inviting the audience to imagine
how they would choose:

Would your choice (for or against treatment) be
influenced by the fact that the hypothetical child I
described has, not cancer but diabetes? We Americans
have been taught to fear cancer, and the first battle in
the war against cancer is against our own attitudes.

The irony is that although John was cured of cancer, he later became a diabetic. He finds more hassles in life from insulin than he ever did from our treatment, more rigidity in lifestyle and no end of the new "chemotherapy" in sight.

I lecture about long-term survivors to each new group of medical students that comes through pediatrics at Yale. I can see from their faces that most of them prefer memorizing the odds that someone will make it than tasting the sweetness of individual victories. "That's very nice, but how representative is that case?"

Not all of them feel that way, though. I watch their faces and can now pick out from their ranks a special type of young person who is being seen in increasing numbers in medical classrooms. Although their classmates cannot tell who they are, I can spot a long-term survivor of childhood cancer five minutes into that lecture.

A Yale undergraduate sat in my office with his eyes downcast. A relative called me to ask if I could speak to Jay. After the boy finished treatment, his parents never again spoke of the experience. Jay grew up sensing that there was a family secret, that he must always bear the mark of a survivor in silence. In college he took a course on Holocaust Literature taught by Elie Wiesel and asks me, "Why did that feel so relevant?"

There were times that Jay tried to ask, but his parents always changed the subject. "Why am I flunking out of college," he asks me without pausing for a response. "God only knows that I'm smart enough and

I want to be a doctor more than anything in the world. But everytime I get in a biology class, my pulse races and my hands become clammy."

For an agonizing hour he poured out his young-ancient soul. Then he rose from the chair with tears pouring down his face. "You're the best doctor I've ever met," he exclaimed. "No one has ever helped me as much as you have. How can I thank you?" I had never gotten to say a word to Jay. I had only listened.

Jay spoke of "being saved for a purpose" and having "passed from death to life." Strange words for a young man whose family was not particularly religious in the usual sense of the word. He left my office without looking back. I didn't hear from him for another year. Then, he reappeared on my doorstep without tears and looked me straight in the eyes. "When I left here, I knew what I had to do. I determined that I wouldn't come back until it was accomplished. I went back to the hospital where I was treated and asked them why they had never anticipated my problems and counseled me. *Why didn't they tell me that I had reason to hope?* But I have to give them credit for their answer."

His doctors said that they had learned from their mistakes and invited him to join them for the summer to interview other survivors. "Be a part of the solution, Jay."

He made his choice. Today Jay is an oncologist himself and speaks to others with cancer about being saved for a purpose.

5

Children Who Chisel

How they cut loose together, David and Yahweh, whirling around before the ark in such a passion that they caught fire from each other and blazed up in a single flame of such magnificence.

Frederick Buechner

*D*ear Crumb-bunny,

I love to watch you playing in your crib when I come to visit. You casually look up at me from your work, remind me that you know that I know that your work matters as much as mine.

I take my breaks, and you do, too. You want to watch boys and girls singing and dancing, so you keep standing and pointing to the TV. For you to "watch" means to take control, climb in front of the video, run it even with your IV hooked up.

Dad lifted you onto the bedside table so you could be in charge. What you can't accomplish for yourself, you assigned to your willing slaves. Neither my work nor Dad's work is more important than these moments of serfdom for you.

You are like little David standing before mighty Goliath. I don't think it even enters your mind that anything could keep you from reaching your goal.

For the past year your parents have kept their eyes on a single goal. There were many potential obstacles in their way, but they never paid them serious attention;

they only concentrated on this bone-marrow transplan-
tation. And they slew a gaggle of giants along the way.

On your honeymoon, perhaps, you could travel to
Florence and see the great statue of David created by
Michelangelo. You giant-slayers should get to know
each other.

      🐾   🐾   🐾

At his request, I visited an adult patient in our
hospital, a man who was bedridden by widespread
cancer. Before his chemotherapy was started, he had
suffered incredible pain that not even morphine could
relieve.

Thanks to effective treatment, the pain was now
under control, but he found the thought of a lifetime of
such drugs overwhelming. He didn't see how he could
face it. He had lost all hope.

In a moment of despair, he cried out, "I wish I
could just end it all with a lethal injection!" A psychiatrist was called, a two-page typewritten note appeared
in the chart testifying to the visit. Oddly (but not so
oddly), he never asked this depressed man what he
believed about death and suicide.

The patient asked to see me because he wanted to
know how my children manage. This question made
me focus on the children, consider things I have come
to take for granted. "Do you believe that the chemotherapy is helping you?" I asked.

"Oh yes!" he replied. "The first day you came to visit me I couldn't even think straight. It was the chemo that took away the pain. I'm not even on morphine now."

"It's not necessary to make a commitment to take chemotherapy for the rest of your life. Start by getting rid of that obstacle. What happens to you for the rest of your life is your choice. Do you think you could handle one cycle?" A cycle of chemotherapy was five days of treatment followed by a three-week rest period.

He looked somewhat relieved but still less than convinced. An intravenous line dripped as we spoke. "Let's break it down further," I proposed. "Can you deal with chemo today?" He nodded vigorously, remembering that his baby daughter would soon come through the door. His day revolved around her visits.

"That is how my patients think of things, in terms of today. One day at a time. Break it down into blocks of time that you know that you can deal with instead of taking on the whole thing now. *Break it down to the hope that you have.*"

"I can do that!" he exclaimed. "One day at a time. Yes, I can do that." That week, he was able to make his choice and remained at peace with it, day by day, for the rest of his life.

There is a story told about the great sculptor Michelangelo. He was once asked how he took a big hunk of marble and turned it into his masterpiece David. His answer, as I recall, was something like this:

"In the marble I saw David, and I chiseled away everything that wasn't David." The artist didn't see the obstacles; he only saw his goal. The obstacles fell away like just so much rubble as he kept his eyes on David.

Occasionally I take a break and sit in the chemo room to see how the children are chiseling away. Often I see a masterpiece come into view. They have such a different view of the world from that of adults, worthy of our attention and consideration. I think about the tools they use and wonder what we as adults can adopt and adapt.

It is not that their obstacles are markedly different from ours. They share our pain and fears, but they do not bear them alone. They tend and feed their important relationships. Children sustain life-giving connections by revealing who they are. No smoke screens here, persona rather than person on display. What you see is what you get. Theologian Paul Minear captures it this way:

> For, to a child, it is more important to be known than to know. The ground of his confidence depends less upon how much he knows about his family than upon the inner awareness that he is known by his family. The psalmist's testimony, "O Lord, thou hast searched me, and known me" (Ps. 139:1), articulates such awareness, an awareness which rises to a climax in the Christian consciousness of being "foreknown," and in the expectation, "Then shall I know fully even as also I was fully known" (1 Cor. 13:12).[13]

These little ones love with an unconditional agape love. I wish that physicians who care for adults had equal access to the sort of love the children bring. They give me the room I need to be the peculiar human being I am. Who I am need not be an obstacle to them.

Relationships are so important to children that they do their best to repair any damage quickly. Their tears quickly point to a relationship at risk. I've had to do many painful things to children over the years, but I've never left a treatment room feeling that the pain was carried away as a grievance. The child's outward expression of pain assists me, poor wretched bumbling adult that I am. I am sure to set things right before the visit ends.

Far more important than the children's opinion of me is their love for their families. Children who die do so without the need for deathbed reconciliations. It is as if their slates are clean. They remind me of the need on a daily basis to set my own accounts straight. They remind me both to ask for and offer forgiveness if I would become a child for the sake of the kingdom of heaven.

Their masterpieces (and the children themselves) are often liberated as Michelangelo's was, by creative imagination. They engage outward talents to tell an inner story. Sometimes I see them retell the story of their cancer in ways that give them power over the marble-like obstacles in their lives.

Rusty symbolizes his cancer as Mount Krebs. He sketches in a multinational counterstrike force against which the tumor cannot hope to prevail. The Red Baron and Snoopy are there, symbolizing the red color of adriamycin and the nurse who massages his shoulders when he is in the hospital. This time Snoopy and the Baron get to work together, partners on Rusty's Dream Team. Group Leader Rusty himself pilots a Sopwith Camel.

Each part of his treatment, every important human and even his dog, are all symbolized in this vintage montage. Mount Krebs shall surely fall! He proudly shows me his work and I note the life-giving light in which he bathes his strike force. There is no darkness here.

Although our powers of creative imagination diminish with age, not even adults are a total loss. If you doubt your abilities, find your own Rusty. Or Ronnie. They will guide your feeble hand.

Ronnie came to us from another hospital in need of further testing, including a bone marrow aspirate. A young colleague learned from the family that their Christian faith was very important to them. He wondered if I could use that to help Ronnie help himself.

I decided to tap Ronnie's creative imagination and suggested that he imagine Jesus in the room helping him. "Think about Jesus. Invite him into the room. When we do something to you, I want you to squeeze Jesus tightly. I also want you to imagine that Jesus is hugging you tightly in return."

Ronnie looked at me as if I was slightly peculiar and then said, "But Jesus is already here." To him, I was overlooking the obvious. The bone marrow went very smoothly.

Ronnie reminds me that all relationships, all imagination find their highest fulfillment in the presence of God who chose to take on flesh like ours and dwell among us. As Leanne Payne says:

> ... to acknowledge the Presence of *the God who is really there* is actually a form of prayer, a way of praying always as the Scriptures exhort us to do. When we do this, the eyes and ears of our hearts are opened to receive the word he is always speaking.[14]

Adults are not without hope. Like Michelangelo, we can chisel away until we cut David loose. Like David, we can dance with Yahweh and catch fire. Like the children, we can blaze up in a single flame of such magnificence that neither life nor death nor anything else in all of creation can separate us from the love of God.

6

Converting a Contract into a Covenant

Love is responsibility of an I for a thou.

Martin Buber

*D*ear Crumb-bunny,
    You are in the last room in the row on the Bone Marrow Unit and cannot see me when I come in. I pause, put on protective shoe covers, chat with visitors. You hear my voice even before you can see me. By the time I come into your view, you extend your little turtle neck, probing out of your shell. You pose and peek and prance in anticipation. Dare I admit how flattered I am?

I watch you smile at me and know that it's not just that you're special to me. I know that I am special to you. How can I begin to describe my relationship to you? I cherish you as well. We met because I am an expert on your rare disease. We all realize today how important it was for you that I do know your disease so well. But we've all grown beyond that day.

How can anyone meet you and just think about diseases, facts, figures, lab results? You smile, you cry, you giggle (the most ordinary of human acts). Performed by you they are acts of rare beauty.

I provide you with my professional services, but a business contract does not adequately describe what we've been through the last year together. We will have to look further for proper words to describe our relationship, mine and thine.

❧   ❧   ❧

Reading the morning paper, you would think that medical practice today is only business and politics. The situation seems utterly without hope.

The public thinks that the doctor-patient relationship isn't what it used to be. Doctors complain that the practice of medicine isn't what it used to be. At least there, we all agree. Things have changed.

There used to be something that made us happier than we are today. We all want the good from the good old days. Here physicians need not muse alone. There are others to share the speculation.

There was a time when Western medical ethics leaned regularly on theological concepts. Ethicist Paul Ramsey calls me back to "the Biblical norm of fidelity to covenant" when he interprets the practice of medicine as one such covenant.[15]

I like that word—*covenant*. But as I read the newspapers and listen to our elected representatives, all I hear are promises to negotiate for a better health-care *contract*. As I listen to the voices of the children, they remind me how the spirit of contracts and covenants so markedly differ. Ethicist William May says:

Contracts are external; covenants are internal to the parties involved. . . . This discussion of contract and covenant, then, forces a return to the world that the biblical covenant presents, as it attempts to deal with the sting of disease, suffering and death.[16]

This understanding points me to the biblical view of covenant and affords the opportunity to redefine the healing partnership between patient and physician. In the Bible there are many opportunities to examine the notion of covenant.

I like the story of Jacob and Laban because it tests the concept of covenant to its limits. The tension focuses on Rebecca, Laban's daughter and Jacob's intended bride. If it were not for the bride, those two men would never have been talking to each other.

Two adults couldn't even agree which language to use when they assembled a group of stones as a "heap of witness" to their agreement. Each used his own language on his sign that marked the site, but they were willing to try because of a common goal that they shared.

Differences in personalities and in conflicts of culture, belief and sense of authority sometimes complicate the ability to live out the doctor-patient relationship as a covenant. We do, however, have a common goal as patients and doctors that makes it worthwhile to stretch toward each other.

José was three years old when a lump proved to be malignant. He received chemotherapy in an effort to avoid radical surgery. When a scan showed that the tumor was growing, we recommended surgery, but the family declined on the advice of a member of their church.

They based their hope on the words of this man who claimed the gift of prophecy that he had a "word from the Lord" that the boy was already healed. Surgery was not needed, he said.

We planned a conference with the parents and asked them to invite the "prophet" and their pastor. As we reviewed the medical facts for them, the church member looked defiant, avoiding eye contact with us, barely listening to our words. The parents gazed in pain and fear at their child. Their pastor listened carefully and asked our opinion about José's chances, with and without the surgery.

"Pastor, everyone in this room is on the same team. We all want José to be healed and we all want to be sure that God is glorified however healing occurs. We'd like you to lead us in prayer for José."

We did not want to pressure the family to accept surgery or to reorient their theology. Our intent was to permit them to face a difficult medical decision, fully informed in a supportive environment where everyone was on their side. Even the "prophet" enthusiastically joined in the most unusual session that has ever been held in my office. We agreed to wait a week and perform another CAT scan. When that showed further tumor growth, surgery was scheduled.

By identifying that which we could share, we found seed for a covenant. In a covenantal relationship, there is the hope for win-win. This process is a form of "second opinion," calling on someone who shared the family's beliefs but could be objective. The pastor was in a better position than they or the church member to discern the difference between prophetic word and noble feeling.

Covenant-fidelity seeks a common ground that transcends individual or institutional authority and points to the perfect love that casts out fear. It does not require that the parties be in perfect agreement on all points, as in a contract.

But it is not always easy to think of the medical intercourse in these terms. Some doctors openly admit feelings of rage and frustration toward unappreciative patients. In an unusually frank essay, one physician expressed a fantasy that many have repressed:

> She tried to bite me. . . . When the people from the diet service came . . . she would either spit at them or hurl a fork or knife their way. . . . My natural urges were to choke her to death. In fact, it gave me a lot of relief to fantasize how I would kill her. . . . Still, every time she was admitted to our hospital, Duchess got from all of us the best of modern medical care.[17]

Anyone who has practiced medicine knows a Duchess. In talking about another "difficult" patient, physician-author Bernie Siegel comes closer to the notion of covenant. He told a woman with breast cancer whose family thought that she was crazy that he loved her.[18]

It is not only difficult to think in a covenantal fashion, it is downright impossible in human terms. The very act of writing about it reminds me how much help I need to carry my part of a covenant forward. And how often I fail.

I sometimes write words like these at night and the next day, come face-to-face with an "impossible" someone I would rather avoid. But then I am reminded of Jesus' words: "Just as you did it to one of the least of these who are members of my family, you did it to me."[19]

Mother Theresa speaks of seeing a Person in a person. With holy eyes, one might even see the Prince of Peace in a Duchess. If it were Jesus himself who was my patient, just how would I go through each step of a painful procedure? With Jesus at my mercy, how much mercy would I show?

It is in relationship to Christ, his covenant with me, and my covenant with him, that mercy guides my hand. With a Person in my clinic, it is a safer place for children.

7

Big Joe and Little Joe

*Schoolboys have no fear of facing
life. They champ at the bit.*

Antoine Saint-Éxupéry

*D*ear Crumb-bunny,
Parents are very important to babies. They can make all the difference in the world to a child. Your mom cares about all the babies and boys and girls she meets. She has a sensitivity to the crises of these others, your spiritual brothers and sisters, and always remembers to pray for them.

This morning Mom asked me about one boy because of her special concern for him. Two floors away on another hospital ward, he had just died. His sudden death was a surprise to us. Somehow, a mother's praying heart had known.

You are your mother's darling and mine as well. Somehow I think that you know that. Doctors aren't supposed to have preferences, but no one begrudges me my special relationship with you.

I brag about you almost more than your mother does. Everyone has to put up with me telling Crumb-bunny stories and my latest dream for you. The teenage patients listen and grin knowingly. They're partial to babies—and dreams too. Then they add, more *solemnly, "I can understand for myself. I've lived. But the babies get to me. They haven't yet lived." They love you, too, and hope and pray for your recovery.*

Someday I would like to introduce you to some of my other favorites. You may crowd out the room, but I think you would all like each other a lot.

ex   ex   ex

It was a shock to open the newspaper and see his picture. To be sure, he must have been proud to be pictured with his ice hockey team. He had hemophilia, and we had advised against contact sports.

He was nine years old then and my concerns were for hemorrhage. But his parents were committed to normalizing his life, so they infused him with concentrate and allowed him to live. They have never regretted that decision.

His mother listened very carefully when several years later we explained about the newly discovered problem of contamination of blood factor concentrate for hemophilia by the agent that caused AIDS. "HIV" had not yet been discovered, nor was there yet a blood test to determine if a blood donor was infected.

Modern concentrates of blood in that era offered a convenient way for hemophiliacs to treat themselves at home. But since they concentrated the blood of many, many donors, they also posed the greatest risk from AIDS. When the blood of single infected donor was pooled with 500 others, it was as if all 500 had been infected.

That year, our best advice was to surrender the freedom that the concentrates of many blood donors provided. Old fashioned "cryo" wasn't as convenient, but it used fewer individual donors to achieve the same dose. Joe made the switch to cryo.

Despite these precautions, eventually Big Joe tested positive for HIV. Four years later, two weeks before Thanksgiving, I was standing by his bed in our Pediatric Intensive Care Unit. A respirator was doing his breathing for him and he was fighting for his life. That was the day he became "Big Joe."

In the bed next to him was another of our team's patients who had just reached the age at which Big Joe had played ice hockey. "Little Joe" had been diagnosed with a rare form of cancer in the same year that we learned that Big Joe was HIV positive.

Despite all our efforts, the cancer kept coming back in his lungs. Now his chest was filling up with fluid, and he could not breathe without help. There was room for no more radiation, and we knew of no other effective treatment. Chest tubes could only drain the fluid for a little while before it would reaccumulate.

Our pediatric surgeons were willing to try to strip off the lining around the lung that seemed to be "weeping" in response to the cancer, but the procedure was risky. He might not come through the operation at all.

Even if he did, he might not be able to breathe on his own and would forever need the use of a respirator.

A brave young boy had made his own decision to try the operation and, characteristically, he survived it. Now our Little Joe, still on a respirator, was bedded down next to our Big Joe. The holiday season did not seem to be off to a promising start.

I have great respect for the special pediatricians who supervise our PICU. In our hospital jargon they are known as "intensivists," and that aptly describes their work. A member of this team approached Big Joe's parents to tell them his grim interpretation of the current findings. The doctor gently probed their feelings about heroic measures and asked if Joe had ever indicated his own preferences.

His mom shook her head when I made my rounds. "This may sound dumb, but I don't think he's going to die this time. He's going to survive this infection. This isn't going to be the one that gets him." There was nothing I could read on the chart to support her optimism. The colleague was right to assume that he might die.

In the next bed it was apparent that recovery from the anesthesia did not mean recovery of independent breathing. Little Joe was still on a respirator and plans were considered to place a "trach" (breathing tube) in his windpipe. There were no sudden success stories in the PICU for our team, no sagas of dramatic recovery.

It was getting tougher and tougher to make those visits to the PICU. One runs out of words and finds oneself fussing with bedside charts and numbers, sharing data rather than feelings. Data don't bite quite so badly.

When you run out of words, it feels safer to round with a team, swooping down on patient and family with your roving band of residents and students. As we approached Big Joe's bed, his mom was reading a small plastic card in front of her. When she saw us coming, she quickly stuffed it in her pocket.

When the others moved on to Little Joe, I lingered behind. "What was that you stuffed in your pocket to hide when we came in?" She blushed and produced a card with a prayer printed on it. "Don't you dare hide anything like that ever again! It's not an either/or matter, medicine and faith."

Little Joe had his trach in place and was not yet able to speak. This made a little man of few words very, very gabby. Except that he was without a voice. So he kept mouthing words and pointing. On his tray table were plaster penguins that he was painting. It was apparent that our Child Life Program had conquered this sanctum sanctorum of technological medicine.

By Thanksgiving Day, even his cousins had invaded. A room next to the PICU became their workshop for the creation of tiny gingerbread houses out of graham crackers, icing, gum drops, and whatever else caught the young architects' fancy. Countertops that are ordinarily littered with ribbons of EKG tracings spewed out by the cardiac monitors were tidied up to become the display case for dozens of these little beauties.

Little Joe's pointing finger became his voice. As nurses and doctors came in, he indicated that each should choose a gingerbread house to take home. It was an honor to carry my new treasure off to my office, happy that Little Joe could divert himself but concerned whether he would ever leave the PICU and the hospital alive.

Big Joe held his own, but there was extensive damage to vital organs. He remained sedated so that he would not fight the ventilator that supported his life. His parents were most often by his bedside, but sometimes I would find his dad visiting with Little Joe and his parents. They had more than a common name and common doctors that bound them together.

Eventually Big Joe woke up as well and both our Joes were transferred to a regular floor to complete their convalescence. Big Joe was the first to make it home. Although he had lost weight during the illness and required a wheelchair until he regained strength, he made a remarkable recovery.

Little Joe remained with us because of the powerful ventilator that he needed. At Christmas his room filled with gifts and new craft projects. Little Joe lived on and began to think about going home even if it was to die. Somehow, the impossible became possible. He and his breathing apparatus moved home where his hospital-based doctors and nurses continued to supervise his care and visit.

Big Joe recovered enough to travel to Europe and return to college. A year later, he is as handsome as ever and full of plans for the future. I saw Big Joe's mom in our clinic once, writing a letter while she waited for her son.

She was carefully choosing her words to write to a PICU doctor. During the crisis, he had asked her about withdrawal of life support. "I want to be constructive," she said, "so that the doctors will learn from the experience how important faith and hope are in determining what happens to these kids. I mostly want to thank him for his excellent care and update him on all that Joe has been able to accomplish during the last year."

I commended her for her intentions and reflected, "Here it is a year later. Who would ever have believed that both Big Joe and Little Joe would still be with us?"

"Little Joe?" she asked with great surprise. "I had no idea that he was still alive. I was always afraid to ask."

"O ye of little faith!" I teased in return.

I look today at Big Joe who is still HIV-positive and Little Joe who still has cancer, and I know what the statistics say. But for a quarter of a century I have been quoting statistics and learning that the human spirit is stronger than any probability. Statistically, neither Big Joe nor Little Joe should be here today. So with them and their parents, I continue to hope.

8

Hearts Unfolding

*God of glory, Lord of love, hearts
unfold like flowers before thee,
opening to the sun above.*

Henry van Dyke

*D*ear Crumb-bunny,
    You are like a flower, little princess. You sit in your laminar air-flow room flirting with me and cooing at your nurses. You love your little tape recorder and keep listening to the words: "Jesus wants me for a sunbeam to shine for him today." You don't just shine, Baby. You dazzle.

    There was a reason I ordered all those baby IQ tests before you were admitted to the Bone Marrow Transplant Unit. I wanted to see if the histiocytes that we found in your brain and spinal fluid had caused any damage. The psychologist called you "precocious" in some areas he tested. He must have offered you a tape recorder to play with.

    Much of what we do in testing babies is to see how you respond to games we adults design. We don't seem much interested or very talented in testing your spiritual development. Even if we were interested, we would probably invent tests to see whether you babies have learned from adults about God and such.

I look at you and feel you embrace me with your smile. I wonder how you would design a test to measure my spiritual IQ.

❧   ❧   ❧

Some time ago, I visited a church in a community where no one knows me. A mother and three children sat down in the pew in front of me, and an eight-year-old carrot-topped girl turned around to greet me. "My father's in the hospital," she declared. "It's his kidney."

I was stunned at first because she had no way of knowing that I was a doctor. Her concern and worry were unmistakable. So I recovered myself and said to her, "Then we'll have to pray for him." She nodded with redheaded vigor.

The worship service opened with announcements that included the sharing of the sort of concern that was burdening this young child. When the pastor asked if anyone had anything to share, her hand shot up. Just as quickly, her mother and older brother grabbed her arm and lowered it.

The announcements came and went without her concerns for her daddy's being raised to the community of faith. The next part of the service was the greeting. As quickly as the pastor invited worshipers to greet each other, my little friend sprang into the aisle, with her hand extended. She covered at least ten rows in the time available, greeting each worshiper with, "My father's in the hospital. It's his kidney."

Of all of the worshipers, only this tender young flower was willing to become vulnerable as she spread her petals and exposed her delicate inner structure in response to heavenly sunshine.

As adults, we seem to have limited expectations of children. We hardly expect them to be *our* teachers. Two millenia ago, when young children saw Jesus and cried out to him in the temple, the adults present became angry. Jesus' response to them was this: "Out of the mouths of infants and nursing babes you (meaning God) have prepared praise for yourself."[20]

I've thought about my little redhead often when I've been in my medical office seeing patients. There are close analogies between her holy vulnerability and that of my patients. In the family of faith, she found a reason to hope. I wonder why her mother did not share her own concern publicly with her faith-family. Surely it was heavy upon her own heart.

Her mother's silence was typical adult behavior. One reason I enjoy my practice with children and young people is that they know how to express themselves. And express themselves they will when adults permit. I was touched a few weeks ago in my own church when the joys and concerns were shared.

A little girl from my own home church was recently diagnosed with leukemia. A school chum of hers stood up in our worship service and asked for prayer for her friend. I tried to imagine how the congregation would have reacted had the pastor or another adult shared the news with us. We were touched not only by the child's illness but by the faithfulness of her little friend.

Out of the mouths of babes. Had God prepared that young girl to prepare us? These were the words of hope that came to my mind, the very words of Scripture on which that part of our liturgy is based:

> Are any among you suffering? They should pray. Are any cheerful? They should sing songs of praise. Are any among you sick? . . . Pray for one another, so that you may be healed. The prayer of the righteous is powerful and effective (James 5:13, 14, 16 NRSV).

Are you really surprised that children can teach us so much? A baby's smile encourages us to unfold our stiff adult petals faster than any reasoned lecture on honesty and transparency can. My little Crumb-bunny helped me and everyone else who visited her in the Bone Marrow Unit shed our protective layers when she laughed at a silly game we played. She was learning new words in those days. As her vocabulary was expanding, part of our daily ritual was to see whose name would be next after *dada* and *mama*. The baby had always heard me called "Dr. Komp," but the letter K is a late sound to be mastered by a baby. Some informality seemed necessary, so I capitalized on her familiarity with *hi*. Our daily ritual was "Hi, Di!"

Nurse Angie was not about to be outwitted. The baby woke up each morning in her life island, calling to any of the nurses standing near the desk. *Aaaaaaah.*

My nemesis-the-nurse insisted that she was saying *Aaaaaangie.*

Then there was the all-important Hanne who would be the one to fly to London to pick up the donated bone marrow. As Crumb-bunny cruised toward the terrible twos, Hanne picked up her nega-tion, *nah,* and repeated it at least once an hour. "Can't you tell?" said Hanne with chin held high. "She's say-ing (Han)ne."

This was our daily game in which our little co-conspirator delighted. *My name first! Return my love with my name on your lips. I would give anything in the world to hear you, blessed child, say my name.*

They didn't teach me to play such games in medi-cal school, but things are changing. When I was a student, there was no place for a future doctor who might weep. There is evidence of hope, even in the "gross" anatomy lab:

> Nervous students in surgical gloves and aprons . . . lined up alongside steel tables where cadavers lay ready for dissection. Instead of feeling pressured to maintain a stoic composure, these first-year medical students were encouraged not to suppress their emo-tions but to cry, laugh, faint, or leave the room if they wanted to. None did, but many said they appreciated the "permission" to do so. . . . "We try to tell them it's okay to feel weird, upset about what they're doing."[21]

At Dartmouth Medical School, former Surgeon General C. Everett Koop has been the catalyst for change toward a different style of mentoring. He and his colleagues hope to inspire future physicians to be more human in their relationships with patients. Such changes in medical education are overdo and might just help resuscitate our mortally ill health-care system.

What would happen to the health care of adults if one highly trained doctor and two super-specialized nurses spent as much time unfolding their hearts the way Angie and Hanne and I did to Crumb-bunny? Could just *one* doctor plead with just *one* adult patient, *Please show me that you love me. Say my name first?* Don't laugh at me. I'm entitled to my dreams. And so are you.

9

The
Apple Doll House
Parables

*No, it was to shame the wise that
God chose what is foolish by human
reckoning.*

1 Corinthians 1:27, 28 (JB)

*D*ear Crumb-bunny,
 I look at Mom looking at you as we talk and I know that you are loved and accepted. Her idea of a perfect Crumb-bunny is just the way you are, and will be.

Someday you'll meet my friend Ruth. Her son, Donny, died ten years ago, but I still think of him in the present tense. Ruth is special because she knows how to value special people. Ruth went to work at the Apple Doll House after Donny died.

The Apple Doll House was a restaurant where some of the weakest and most vulnerable members of our community could come and work and hold their heads high.

I watch you, my little love, and note that you are one of the wise ones. I know that when you grow up, you will have a heart for God's most fragile creatures.

ഇ ഇ ഇ

We have no idea yet what causes most cases of cancer in children. For most, it happens without warning. Not so for some of my most special patients, children with Down's syndrome. Their abnormal chromosome can lead to cancer as well as birth defects. Morris West calls them the "clowns of God."[22]

Leukemia is their most common malignancy, but other tumors happen as well. What distinguishes the Down's child with cancer from others in my practice is that their parents come so well-prepared. Oddly enough, I find that these special children have also been my most valued teachers.

During my training, we were advised to recommend institutionalization to families of retarded children. Now, most of them grow up in their families, supported by regional centers. And some of these regional centers are extra, extra special.

The Apple Doll House Restaurant in my hometown is closed now and its building is used for other worthy purposes. Its former enterprises have been relocated to a more spacious restaurant that offers more job opportunities for retarded adults. It was in this restaurant that some of my fondest memories took shape.[23]

I had a phone call one day from a man who identified himself as a computer specialist. His teenage son with Down's syndrome had undergone surgery for cancer and they hoped to find the right doctor to coordinate his further care.

His surgeon thought that an adult oncologist would be appropriate since it was an adult-type tumor in an adult-sized person. But Down's syndrome had complicated Rodd's entire life. His parents could not believe that their son should be managed like the average adult.

Rodd's father used his own expertise to shop among pediatricians for the "right" doctor. Although he had never sought for someone with special expertise in cancer in Down's syndrome, my name kept appearing on other computer programs he used. "But who told you about my special interest in Down's syndrome?" I asked. I had never published anything on the subject. My "expertise" is defined by my love for God's special clowns.

"Then we really were 'sent' to you!" he replied. "I didn't even know that."

Rodd's tumor never returned, but we kept in frequent touch because of mutual respect and unrivaled fun. He would even agree to a barium enema if I curtsied properly and called him "Your Lordship."

Rodd is witty, active, and proud and would dance me off my feet at his birthday parties if I didn't plead middle age and propose a younger partner. Praise the Lord for amazing Grace. His girlfriend, who also has Down's syndrome, can dance all night.

We met at Apple Doll House. This time, he was my guest. Mary Kate, the senior hostess, came to take our orders. As His Lordship perused the menu, he sneaked a glimpse of this wondrous creature out of the corner of his eye. All the dining-room staff that day were adults with Down's, and Rodd thought he was in heaven when he saw who was running the place.

As Mary Kate glided away from the table with our orders, Rodd permitted himself a cautious sideward glance then returned his attention to us. He shook his head contemplatively and said, "Stunning woman!"

Mary Kate returned with our desserts and the check. As we were leaving the Apple Doll House, his mother asked, "Rodd, what do you think of this place?" He looked around him and said wistfully but clearly, "It's wonderful to see so many handicapped people."

Do you think it's wonderful when you see many handicapped people? We, the clever, are often the ones who are handicapped. And definitely lacking in imagination. One young man I know with severely impaired speech is in love. His sweetheart, who is deaf, taught him sign language and she "hears" only the beautiful fluency of his hands.

The miracle of grace continues. Linguists in California are getting very clever with those affected by faulty speech. They find that some persons with Down's syndrome are freed to express themselves quite poetically by the keyboard of a computer. A teenager named Christine chose to write about God and turned to the researcher to say, "He's gonna like this." I'm sure she's right: "I like God's finest whispers."[24]

Because of a major birth defect, Rev. Harold Wilke lacks the hands to execute sign language, but he has the most talented toes in the United Church of Christ. Karl Menninger quotes Wilke: "I can't shake hands with you ... I never had hands ... I was expected by my parents to do everything my brothers did, and I learned alternative ways—toes instead of fingers."[25]

Do you hope to see many handicapped, special people? It is not only society at large and the health-care system that may fail them. Historically, the religious community has not done much better. Reverend Wilke would not always have been considered candidate material for ordained ministry.[26]

Do you, like Rodd, find it wonderful or is your first impulse to run? Sometimes we run in our hospitals, and even in our houses of worship. We may not exclude the mentally and physically handicapped by policy, but the clever seem chronically lacking in imagination. Without holy imagination, we are not a people of hope.

What response can we make to what is weak and foolish, common and contemptible by human reckoning? We can become a caring society if we examine our impulses and stop running. We are a healing community when we use a thousand tongues and fingers and toes to repeat God's finest whispers.

10

A Matter
of Life and Death

*Life is serious all the time, but living
cannot be ... You may have all the
solemnity you wish in your neckties,
but in anything important (such as
sex, death, and religion), you must
have mirth or you will have
madness.*

G. K. Chesterton

*D*ear Crumb-bunny,
    A bone-marrow ward is a place to think about life and death. All the patients are here because they desperately want to live but not everybody will walk out the door. No one knows better than the doctors and nurses who work here what it means to contemplate life and death in the same thought, capture their essence in the same breath.

You babies who have come here as patients have taught us much. You know what it means to be vulnerable but trusting, dependent but not depressed. That's a hard lesson but a necessary one for adults to relearn.

There are older kids and adults in this hospital who must sometimes wear a diaper. But unlike you, they weep when they soil, and someone else must come to change them. They are very proud people, as Jesus knew.

The Christian story says that God partook in our experience, shared that tension on the edge of life and death. God was diapered in Bethlehem, learned to say Abba in a carpenter's shop. And when he had profound *lessons to share with adults about life and death and pride, he pointed to someone like a little Crumb-bunny.*

You are a teacher, little one, someone who has with a message for us all.

୫   ୫   ୫

When a child comes to our wards with the diagnosis of cancer, someone may ask whether the patient knows that he is dying. But cancer is a word, not a sentence. Cancer is easier to heal than a morbid fear of cancer.

Vulnerable children have taught me not to fear fear itself. From the children and their parents I have learned that not all fear of cancer should be avoided. Fear can alert us to danger. It only becomes noxious when our response, our fear of our fear, prevents us from moving in life-affirming ways.

If I feel a lump in my breast, fear that it is cancer can move me in one of two directions. It can move me to a doctor for early diagnosis and treatment. Or fear can lead to procrastination and denial, propose fantasies and inertia. If fear compels me to act, it is my friend.

"I have a terminal illness," says Peter Kreeft. "You are invited to read [his book *Love Is Stronger Than Death*] for the same reason. . . . Life is always fatal. No one gets out of it alive."[27] Someone with cancer is no more 'terminal' than the rest of us, nor are they to be subjected to pitiful pity.

In the adult world, one of the greatest impediments to conquering cancer is delay in diagnosis. A false kind of hope spins tales to the psyche. This is rarely seen with children. The typical child I see for cancer is brought to a doctor the same day the first symptom is recognized. This is an important reason that we have made so much progress in their care.

The Big C. The biggest fear. A person with cancer is no more "terminal" than the rest of us. Such toxic fear takes on magical qualities in some of the most rational, non-magical thinkers I know. I see this force at work when I meet people for the first time and the conversation turns to the usual small talk. When I say that I am a pediatric oncologist, I wait for the automatic small step backward, away from me. My patients know this fear as well, that our proximity might hex them or someone they love.

Once when I was shopping, an almost-voiceless friend sought my medical opinion. She showed me an antibiotic that remained on her bathroom shelf after a previous illness. She was suffering from laryngitis and wondered if these capsules would help. This particular medicine does nothing for viral infections and can have undesirable side effects. I recommended against her taking it.

Another customer overheard our conversation. He had no idea who I was but thought he certainly had more expertise than a middle-aged woman in shorts and a T-shirt. "That antibiotic can do you no harm," he disagreed without being consulted, and my friend asked him if he was a doctor. No, he was a dentist.

She thought she should clarify who I was. "That woman with whom I was talking, she's a medical doctor. She is an oncologist."

"Oncologist!" he exclaimed, assuming I was out of earshot. "Do you know what that means? All her patients are terminal. Why, that's pitiful!"

We tend to divide life from death, living from dying, as if they happened to two different sets of people. With the dying we place all those with cancer. An experience reminds me how difficult it is to think of life and death at the same time. I was leading a group of physicians and clergy who came together to explore a common interest in physical and spiritual wholeness. A hospital chaplain expressed his desire for better communication with his medical friends. "The way I see it," he explained, "doctors should let the clergy know when someone is dying. That is where your job ends and ours begins." His statement captured my full attention. He startled me.

Some physicians flee the bedsides of the dying as if we ourselves are not safe. When we do, we leave a gap, forsaking the sufferer. It was this gap that the chaplain saw. But did he not leave another one in its place? I would have thought that he, like Jesus, might have something to offer the living as well as the dying. As I understand it, the Christian gospel, which the chaplain was ordained to proclaim, is good news.

The chaplain saw his job and mine as serial rather than parallel, independent rather than interdigitating. My responsibility and the hope that I can bring does not end with the last prescription. To keep the covenant, I must address my own fear of cancer, my own fear of death, and move back to the bedside. "Til death us do part," a covenantal promise, would make a more appropriate summary statement for a doctor-patient relationship. And that is not bad news. It is a reason to hope.

"Peace I leave with you," said Jesus. "My peace I give to you. I do not give to you as the world gives. Do not let your hearts be troubled, and do not let them be afraid."[28] This peace he speaks of is more than the absence of fear. It is a gift from Christ for those who make the choice. *Do not let your hearts be troubled* is a command, not a suggestion, a choice we can all make. And that is good news indeed.

To participate in the healing of others, we ourselves must do something about our own wounds. We need to start with our ideas about life. For some bizarre reason, we think that we are already experts about life and that it is only death that holds the unknown. The grim statistics on failed marriage, unwanted pregnancy, dysfunctional families, and social despair cry out that we have much as a society to learn about life. We need valid reasons to hope.

Since the publication of Elisabeth Kübler-Ross's book, *On Death and Dying*, some have said that death has come "out of the closet."[29] Dying seems to have found a way to separate itself from living, to take on, so to speak, a life of its own.

We can learn much about life, healing, and hope from those who work with the dying. Shiela Cassidy, a British hospice physician, says that she has a "very expensive ringside seat at the fight" but concludes:

> We have a duty to report back the truth of what we see: that the facts are friendly; that the blind see, the lame walk, the lepers are cleansed, and the good news is proclaimed to the poor—that the kingdom of God is among us, and that herein lies our hope.[30]

A few years ago a close friend struggled with widespread cancer. On a drive to Boston following a chemotherapy cycle, we made many emergency stops. Each time Ginnie returned, she looked a bit wearier and a lot paler. I would resume driving without comment, until the next stop.

One time, she got back in the car, looked up at me with a mischievous little-child grin to say, "This is going to sound very corny. The Big C isn't cancer. The Big C is Christ." For her, no disease would be allowed to take on power in her life. Cancer would not have the last laugh. In choosing to make Christ the center of her life, Ginnie could face cancer, chemotherapy, and even death itself. In making that choice, she was healed of the fear of cancer and the fear of death.

Not many months later, the tumors in her body were growing and it was time to invite hospice into her home. She called me at work many times to say, "Tell your patients, hospice is about life."

Christ is the Big C. Hospice is life. These statements do not ignore mortality. They simply put cancer and death in their proper perspective. In Christ and with hospice, Ginnie found that she would never be alone or abandoned. She was free to live and laugh.

In some Greek communities, Christians gather the day after Easter to tell each other jokes, honoring God's greatest joke that took place on Easter morn.[31] But the healing property of humor is lost if we don't get the joke, fail to understand the punch line.

> When this perishable body puts on imperishability, and this mortal body puts on immortality, then the saying that is written will be fulfilled: "Death has been swallowed up in victory.[32]"

A friend told me that in his family the members whose lives have been touched with cancer have the best sense of humor. I can understand this. It is children with cancer who taught me hilarity, to risk laughing when the world might dictate tears. One child tells me that it is when I laugh that he knows he has hope.

In reaching my hand to the plastic window that separates Crumb-bunny from me, I delight in her delight of me. We do not let out hearts be troubled. We both have a terminal illness, she and I, but we have a reason to hope. *Where, O death, is your victory? Where, O death, is your sting?* She giggles and I giggle, sharing our Easter hilarity. We both understand God's greatest joke.

11

Risen with Healing in His Wings

*Life and light to all he brings, risen
with healing in his wings.*

Charles Wesley

*D*ear Crumb-bunny,
      The statistics say that you have no hope to survive. You will die, they say, that all my medical miracles will not avail. Because of those statistics, I am reaching beyond what is familiar, and the reach is wider than some suspect.

      Does Dr. Grandma pray for you to be healed? Baby, you had better believe it. Someone very wise summarized our journey together, yours and mine: "Work as if everything depends on you and pray as if everything depends on God." Your doctor is into combined modality therapy.

      Some people believe there never were any miracles. Other people believe that there were only miracles during the time that the Bible was being written and then they stopped. Still others think that God only works miracles independent of medical intervention. The arguments are without end. Personally, I think some of those people are well meaning but a little bit confused.

I have lived too long and seen too much to tie you up in tidy intellectual knots. Because I hope, my princess, I work and pray for you to be healed.

૨ઢ   ૨ઢ   ૨ઢ

It was one of those collegial but challenging conferences where physicians of different disciplines exchanged ideas on difficult tumor cases. The case at hand was that of a baby who had broken all the rules.

"Are you sure you had the right diagnosis?" asked the radiotherapist of the pathologist. "I've never seen this particular tumor respond that way. You must be wrong."

"No, I'm not wrong!" responded the somewhat indignant pathologist. "I know that tumor when I see it."

"Well, maybe you want to look at it again."

"Looking at it again isn't going to change the diagnosis!'"

The radiation therapist looked elsewhere for an explanation of the unexplainable and turned to the chemotherapist managing the case. "That chemotherapy must have done the job."

"Don't look over here for the explanation. We only used a radio-sensitizing dose. Besides, the tumor was growing through the last course of different drugs. Are you sure it wasn't the radiation therapy that did the job?"

"No way. This tumor has never gone away like that before." He turned half-joking to the radiologist who had interpreted the scans. "Are you sure those are the right films?"

"Yes, they're the right X-rays! You can tell from the comparison to the old ones that it's the same child. Only the tumor is gone."

"It doesn't make sense," the radiation therapist kept repeating.

The minutes of that conference simply reflected the lack of a known medical explanation for the disappearance of the tumor. The medical minutes did not reflect other activities on her behalf. Teams from a local church fasted and prayed daily for Bethany, two by two. Many other family friends prayed for her tumor to go away.

ʘ ʘ ʘ

These days if the word *healing* is used in conjunction with health, it is most often interpreted to reflect some activity other than medical practice. Several years ago, I had lunch at a Trappist monastery with a former brother of that community. Before lunch we attended a service with the brothers and other guests. During the prayers of the people, my companion asked prayer for, "My friend Di, and her ministry of healing."

At lunch, several fellow-guests asked me about my "ministry of healing." They were shocked to learn that I am a medical doctor. They did not expect a "healer" to be a medical doctor. Personally, I am not comfortable with the term "healer" for any human person. There is a sign over a mission hospital that summarizes it all for me: *We treat; Jesus heals.* I simply cooperate. I am part of God's combined modality team.

"I have a brilliant idea how to reduce Francesca's side effects," I proudly announced to a mother. For months her child's blood counts had dipped dangerously low, and now I had an idea how to avoid that problem.

"You and your brilliant ideas!" sassed her mother in return. "Some of us parents have been talking. We pray and then you get your brilliant ideas. Just don't take all the credit!" Her blood counts never reached the danger level again.

૩ઢ   ૩ઢ   ૩ઢ

"My miracle man!" was the greeting of a cardiologist who brought Mike back from the jaws of death when he removed a clot from a vital coronary artery. Days earlier when I joined my friend's family and pastor in the coronary care unit, the "miracle man" was in shock and dying. As the medical team was preparing to take Mike for a final attempt to save his life, we were praying (against the odds) for his recovery.

A nurse moved toward our circle but the doctor held her back. "Don't interrupt them," he said quietly. "They are praying." The same nurse called my office an hour later to say, "It's a miracle. He's out of shock. We can hardly believe it."

☙   ☙   ☙

The families I just described all have an active concept of healing. But what would they think if they consulted me in my medical office and I said, "I am sure that I can heal your child?" They would probably run out the door to find themselves a "real" doctor. Patients expect a different vocabulary from a medical specialist who fits squarely within traditional Western medicine. But the three families I described have not placed all their hope in imperfect scientists.

What if Mike has another heart attack? How will Francesca's family react if their daughter's future life is not one of perfect health? What will all those praying people think if Bethany has only a remission and not a cure of her malignancy?

I worry about people whose faith is based on their ability to get God to perform on command. The families I describe and their friends are not such people. They have met other faithful families whose loved ones have not survived and have seen the healing presence of God in their lives despite their losses. The world is a richer place for the journeys that they've all traveled.

The adults in these stories have come into a relationship with God that cannot be changed by subsequent medical events. The whole work of God is displayed in their lives for they themselves have been healed.

Are these stories miracles of divine healing or miracles of modern medical science? All of these families involved were convinced of a spiritual element in their loved one's improved health. But they were equally convinced of the value of modern medical care and continue to comply diligently with all orthodox medical recommendations. For them it is not an either/or matter. Neither is it for me.

Never far behind the question about divine healing are questions about divine reasons why children suffer. Jesus was asked one day by his own friends. "Who sinned, this man or his parents, that he was born blind?"[33] His answer was quite simple: "Neither this man nor his parents sinned." Parents tormented by imagined guilt think that the answer to their offspring's cancer is who. And the "who" must be themselves.

Jesus took clay from the earth, mixed it with his own saliva and put it on the man's eyes "so that the work of God might be displayed in his life."[34] Jesus converted *why* and *who* into *what*. I feel compelled to do the same.

᠊᠊᠊   ᠊᠊᠊   ᠊᠊᠊

"Do you believe in healing?'" asks a young mother, and I know in my heart that she is not asking if I believe that the chemotherapy I just gave her baby will work. And if she is anything like other mothers, she is wondering why her baby got cancer—if she herself is in some way responsible.

I move past the why and the who and consider what I can offer the young woman's baby, not only from modern medicine but also from God. I know that if that medical treatment has not worked for all such infants, it has worked for many. I cannot hold back from recommending it for her son because it hasn't worked every time. The same holds true for prayer.

I will not hold back from asking for God's personal healing touch on her baby because other children have died despite earnest prayer. I have seen the unexpected too often. Nor will I ask God to make a clear distinction between my work and his. My work is his as well. But I suggest to Naomi that she put every facet of her life, not just the baby's tumor, in God's hands and to invite her husband to join her as well.

As a physician, I will work as hard as I can in a profession with an honorable history. As a Christian I will also pray as hard as I can in a religious tradition that I also hold to be honorable. Children need to be healed. So do the rest of us.

12

Beauty
by Proximity

To keep beauty in its place is to make all things beautiful.

George Santayana

*D*ear Crumb-bunny,
   From your life island you smile invitingly,
pleased when I come up against your window.
You reach your pudgy little hand toward me and then
play your tape recorder again. When the song is complete, you remove the cassette and unravel the tape.
Then you laugh and look to Mom for approval.

   Since the day that you started your treatment, you
have been a very busy baby. Your hospital visit days
were packed full. You ate and slept and flirted and
modeled one of your many prissy little dresses.

   I think you were born knowing you were a girl-
baby. Your idea of a wardrobe is a frock a day. Have
you ever worn the same outfit twice? I think you will
be a bit vain when you grow up. Vain, perhaps, but
very beautiful. Since you're a baby, we'll allow such
righteous vanity!

   Don't stop there when it comes to beauty, little
friend. You come from a family of heart-beautiful
people.

Learn what you can from staying close to Mom and Dad. Then, my dear, you will truly be beautiful.

🐌   🐌   🐌

"You know, it's all in the make-up and lighting,'" the photographer offered as he tried to get his subject to relax for the camera. "You wouldn't even recognize most of the top models outside the studio." *Life* magazine had sent him to my home to transform a middle-aged academic into proper pictorial material.

I adjusted the collar of my dress to hide my second chin. "Don't worry about that," he encouraged. "I can take care of that." He was visibly relieved when my Yorkshire Terrier climbed into my lap. To the photographer's delight, Ashley started posing without being coached. "He's great!" he exclaimed and then carefully added, "You're not bad yourself."

The conversation ultimately turned to world-famous beauties. Most beautiful women make it hard for the other people in the same photo, devastating them by comparison. Princess Di, on the other hand, is not only beautiful herself, she makes other people look good as well. Her shy smile enhances how we perceive her companions. When she weeps, we see her companions naked, as they are without her presence.

Finally the photographer called, "It's a wrap!" and he indicated to his assistant which film rolls to mark with a star. These were the shots when the dog was at his best. Hopefully, Doctor Di had been suitably beautified by proximity.

This "beauty by proximity" is something I see each day in a clinic where bodies have been seemingly ravaged by disease and treatment. We used to have a sign in our clinic that said, "Bald is beautiful." And years ago another one said, "Thank you, Kojak." Today it's Michael Jordan we adore.

One of my four-year-olds said years ago, "It's what's on a person's inside that counts." She knew how beautiful she was and allowed you (if you were nice) to stroke her shiny bald head.

When the head must be covered, fashionable headgear is a popular alternative for the kids. One mother designed a railroad engineer's cap for her daughter out of a patchwork of leftover fabric. Soon, every girl in her school had to have a similar hat. In that school, Barbara set the new standard for beauty. Long after she completed her treatment and her hair grew back, she and her classmates were still wearing these caps.

The more time I spend with these children, the more contagious I find their beauty of the heart. There is one advantage to not having hair—their eyes draw our own and become their focal feature.

The eyes are invariably eloquent, mirroring the heart and health. After their hair grows back, I still find myself drawn first to their eyes. For patients, the doctors' eyes are important as well. It is to our eyes rather than our words that they turn to measure truth and hope.

Years ago I explained to a father that his four-year-old daughter would lose her hair. He asked if it would not be better to leave her leukemia untreated and simply let her die. Fifteen years later, she is a college student, cured of leukemia. I still see her eyes first and don't even notice her hair.

Oh, I know it is there, fully regrown, but for the life of me I would be hard-pressed to tell you what color it is. But her eyes, yes, her eyes are an impish blue framed by long lustrous lashes. She looks boldly into my eyes, challenging me to explore her very soul.

Many physicians freely admit that they choose other areas of medicine because they do not want to be near the suffering of children. They worry if pediatrics will engender constant concern for the welfare of their own families. They know that even children suffer and die. Sometimes they fear the consequences, should one little one look into their very soul.

Similarly, many young physicians assume that our oncology clinic must be the most depressing assignment that they will face during their training. Most of them are unprepared for the opportunities for self-beautification. Some kids are more direct than others in their efforts to improve upon the rough-hewn humans who are their caregivers. I warned an intern one day before we knocked to see if Marnie was ready for examination.

"How many times do I have to tell you!" Marnie said, sadly shaking her head at me in disapproval. "You use the wrong shade of 'Loving Care.' You can still see the gray. There's absolutely no reason for you to look this old."

"But Marnie, I *am* this old. Middle age isn't a disease," I lamely protested.

"You don't act old. Why should you look so old?" retorted this pert teenager. "Gray hair is for people like my mother."

"Motherhood isn't a disease either. Besides, I'm older than your mother."

"Next time I come back, I expect to see no visible gray hair." That was her final pronouncement. It is a fearful thing to fall into the hands of a living teenager.

Marnie herself is a beautiful girl who was coping creatively with the changes that chemotherapy imposed on her young body. A carefully chosen wig disguises her baldness, and skillfully applied make-up enhances her lovely features. She is impatient with me when I wear my trifocals instead of contact lenses and pay more attention to my paperwork than to my appearance.

This self-assured young woman who cheerfully greets everyone when she walks into the chemotherapy room is far different from the teenager I met months ago. The diagnosis of cancer and its aftermath accentuated a sadness she had experienced for many years. Ironically, it was in this oncology clinic that she herself was bequeathed beauty by proximity.

Competent care involves more than the application of scientific principles and protocols. We were fortunate to have a nursing assistant as a member of our team who brought out the beauty of all those whose lives she touched. Esther cradled many a teenager as we performed bone marrow aspirates and spinal taps as part of their treatment.

"You're my baby," I would hear her purr. "If I hold you, nothing bad can happen to you." When Marnie needed to share something painful with me, she confided in me from the safety of Esther's arms.

When we first met Marnie, she had no idea how beautiful a person she was on the inside. Coached by Esther, she learned her own worth. That beauty now radiates from the inside and touches all members of our extended family who have the good fortune to meet her.

Am I contradicting myself to simultaneously speak of physical and inner beauty? Not at all. For a young woman with cancer like Marnie, we must sometimes restore the sense of physical beauty before the beauty of the heart can shine through. Programs such as "Look Good/Feel Good" through the American Cancer Society recreate beauty from ashes, self-esteem from side-effects. More than most women, they learn that beauty is not just skin deep.

In a sense, all cancer patients experience a sort of new birth. So often I hear the biblical phrase "passed from death to life" from them. They are often reduced to a state of vulnerability that they have not experienced since their birth. And for most, they become bald as the day they were first born.

They must learn from those of us around them how they are perceived and valued in this world. If it is reasonable to tell Crumb-bunny how beautiful she is, to feed her righteous baby vanity, then the woman (or man) with cancer deserves no less. Whether stroking a shiny bald head or enjoying a thick new pelt, touch can make someone beautiful as well.

But how do we, the healthy, get beautified? We can choose the people whom we allow to influence us, seek those who can teach us life's most profound lessons. But there are risks. Jesus puts it this way, "Those who find their life will lose it, and those who lose their life for my sake will find it."[35]

If we wish to find out what life is all about, we had best not run from those people who threaten us. For me it was children with cancer. For you, there may be a different lovegiving, lifesaving embrace.

"Happy are they who bear their share of the world's pain," says Jesus. "In the long run they will know more happiness than those who avoid it."[36] It is more painful to stand at a "safe" distance than to be right there in the thick of it. The closer I am to these children, the more likely I am to be transformed by their radiance. By the time that I retire, I expect to be a very beautiful woman.

13

The Color of Pain

*God whispers to us in our pleasures
. . . but shouts in our pains: it is his
megaphone to rouse a deaf world.*

C. S. Lewis

*D*ear Crumb-bunny,
  Today is not one of your good days. Your poor mouth has ulcers, and your little bum is so raw that you wail when you pee. I hate to see you cry like that.

Your misery reminds me of all the painful tests I've had to do on you over the last year. Your little mouth used to collapse into a frown when you saw me come in the room. I think of all the ways that I cope with your pain and what it is that keeps me from running out of the room.

I face your pain by getting into my can-do medical mode, dial up the dose of morphine, look ahead to when the sores will heal. I know that just like the bone marrows and the spinal taps, even this pain is just for a season. But do you?

Your mom comes right along when I do anything painful to you. She and I chatter and think about how important the test is rather than what it takes to do it. Years from now when you are safe, we'll lose our need *to chatter and laugh. But today, we must get you (and us) through.*

You whimper in your sleep and I want to take your pain away forever and hurl it off this planet. What color for you is the color of pain?

❧   ❧   ❧

In our clinic, everything painful seems relative and each of us has our own way of coping. Most of our young friends are perfectly clear about the rank order of owies. There are finger-sticks and spinals. And then there's the dreaded bone marrow. Nobody likes a bone marrow.

Dip a brush in a pot of paint of as bold a shade of red as you can imagine. Hot tomato isn't a bad choice. Neither is crimson blaze. But blood-red. Ah, yes. Especially blood-red would make the point nicely.

Don't chintz in the sweep of your brush or the intensity of the shade if you want to be properly descriptive. Dracula blood-red. Start your sanguineous stroke where the hip bone's connected to the tail bone and then sweep over to the thigh bone, painting back and forth in radiating ruby rings.

This is pain that we're describing. When we're talking about the pain of a bone marrow, we should be suitably graphic if we would tell the truth. Sometimes the experience of pain can be expressed in words or colors. For severe pain, children see red.

Those of us whose job it is to prevent or alleviate

the pain of children have the extra challenge to try to understand pain in their terms. We dare not think that a child's viewpoint is the same as ours.

Youngsters rarely think of medication as the solution for pain in a cause-and-effect manner. Their hope for pain relief comes on from a more personal considerations. Psychological pain cannot be easily separated from the physical experience of a medical procedure.

There is an adage in pain-management circles that goes like this: "Pain is what the person with pain says it is." As a physician who must sometimes inflict pain on children, I am compelled to understand the length and breadth and height of pain from a child's point of view. I must posit myself with them if would help them with their distress.

Numerical scales are quantitative ways for clinicians to ask older children and adults to describe their pain. "On a scale of 1 to 10," we ask, "how would you rate your current pain?" On this scale, 1 is no pain and 10 is the worst pain you can imagine. If I were a four-year-old, all misery would be a 10. We call these kids our Sarah Heartburns, and we know more than a few little Sarahs.

Sarah comes to the treatment room tearfully and verrrrrrrrrry slowly. Her thousand quasi-logical excuses en route might appeal to a very naïve parent, or pathetically young doctor, but we all lost our innocence long ago. Sarah knows that, so she holds back her trump card.

"Ah, Sarah!" I greet her, oozing with friendliness. "Hop right up here." She has gnawed her favorite security blanket threadbare so her mom makes a fast swap for number-two alternate from her Big Brown Bag. As our nurse's aide Esther lifts the child to the examining table, Sarah launches another small stall. I dare not let her catch me looking at my watch or I am dead meat.

I glove and paint Sarah's backside an iodine-rich brown. I am ready to start, a syringe of numbing Lidocaine loaded and lifted. Sarah murmurs, "I gotta pee."

I snicker and Sarah's tone becomes strident. "It's not funny. I *really* mean it." Too late, I try to abort a second-wave snicker rising in my throat, but she hears it and releases a warm stream of golden revenge.

Esther strips away the soaked surgical toweling and Sarah's undies. Mom pats her bag, locating the fresh change of clothing she always brings for the child. As I reglove to start over, Sarah warns, "Don't forget to say 1-2-3!" To control the controller is to control the pain.

ॐ   ॐ   ॐ

A portion of Sarah's pain is the sadness with which her mother anticipates the procedure. Parents dread the possible test results as much as the instruments that invade their babies' tender flesh. We learned a valuable lesson about the actual physical pain of a bone marrow a few years ago.

One of our partners planned a research project that needed bone marrow from normal volunteers. A laboratory co-worker frequently volunteered. She was paid handsomely for her pain and always seemed prepared to donate again.

Our volunteer was able to control her own date with destiny, her certain knowledge that she did not have to think of bone-marrow aspirates as part of the rest of her life. She was not concerned how her bone marrow might look under the microscope, whether leukemia had relapsed. Her hope lay in her paycheck, not in the results. She was not at risk. She was sure and in control, and that is the way we prefer our lives to be.

In the course of my work, I frequently provide a second opinion for parents whose children are under treatment at other medical centers. In many cases, the recommendations of the first doctor were entirely appropriate and I wonder why the parents traveled so far to have their questions answered.

They have made the trip to rid themselves of pain. Sometimes I can relieve them by listening patiently to questions: Why was that scan done? My son was so frightened being in that cold room by himself. Why was such a powerful medication given to so small a child? By honoring their need and right to know, I fill a yawning chasm that has been packed with their pain.

I see the relief registering on their faces. But not all parents.

Some parents may seek to ease their pain by searching for someone who can eliminate all uncertainty. The comment of one mother with great mental anguish helped me see this more clearly.

ᔒ ᔒ ᔒ

Susan's daughter was first thought to have a highly lethal form of cancer. Had that diagnosis been correct, Tiffany would need surgery, chemotherapy, and radiation according to a prescribed protocol. That treatment would be rough on the child but it most likely would have been curative.

Rather than cancer, Tiffany has a benign disease that may well go away on its own. Surgery, radiation or chemotherapy can be held in reserve and are unlikely to be needed. After several months of living with this benign but uncertain situation, Susan admitted that she was jealous of the parents in the same clinic whose children had cancer.

She (almost) wished that her daughter had certain malignancy rather than an uncertain future. It might even be easier to know that Tiffany will surely die than not to know how the story will end. Susan was not in control of her daughter's future, her own angst. She was seeing red. She was searching for someone who knew all the answers about her daughter's disease. Then, and only then, could she begin to relinquish control, learn the lessons of trust and uncertainty, to let go of her pain.

All worthwhile human relationships, whether with loving friend or respected physician, can only hint of a better way to trust. A wise man once said, "Trust in the LORD with all your heart, and do not rely on your own insight. In all your ways acknowledge him, and he will make straight your paths."[37]

As long as we keep seeking answers in ourselves or others to mollify our pain, we will fall back into the fear of uncertainty. There is a tension in trust, the knowledge that we must learn to trust and be trustworthy. Although a physician, I am only human, not much more certain than Susan. Parents and doctors alike, we must seek Someone worthy of our full trust, especially when the future is uncertain.

❧ ❧ ❧

When I think about pain, I remember the heartbreak of a young mother and father listening to a diagnosis, prognosis, implications for their future. But this couple, Crumb-bunny's parents, moved past their pain, fought back. They armed themselves with a notebook, tape recorder, and telephone—parental tools of the medical martial arts. There were times that I was overwhelmed by their questions. But then I remembered that this was indeed war. I had hundreds of patients to care for and they had one surviving child.

Let them fight their good fight. *For once, Di, be a simple foot-soldier instead of a general.*

Most parents who seek my advice are like these young parents and that is good. They master the art of advocacy for their children in ways that forge a healthy link with their doctors and fortify their other relationships. But on occasion, there is another sort of parent. Not fighters but flighters, they are running from even their necessary pain.[38]

❦   ❦   ❦

Cindy told me the case history without seeming to notice that her child was destroying my office. Her husband broke in often to correct her, all petty points. Mother and father talked at the same time, vied for my attention as their son, unregarded, vied for theirs. While the parents paralleled their monologues, Ricky used a red Magic Marker to spell out his pain on my white file cabinets, inscribing four-letter words that no four-year-old child should know how to spell.

There were only two points on which the parents seemed to converge. Rage ignited as Cindy talked about the first pediatrician. "Dr. High N. Mighty," she hissed. "He thinks he is God Almighty!"

Jack released his death-grip on his briefcase as he nodded in vigorous agreement with his wife for the first time. Their mutual hatred for this man, the tenuous glue that holds their fragile marriage together, is their single impetus to dialogue. Before the illness, it was the child himself who kept them together as a family.

With the threat to Ricky's life, they scramble to maintain their equilibrium. They'd scrambled thousands of miles that day to my office. If I fail to bellow their rage, I will be sending them away with less than they came for.

Jack opened his briefcase. His voice softened as he made a votive offering to me—a sheaf of publications about his son's disease, all from my pen. "You've written everything important that there is to say," he pleaded as he reached for his wife's hand. "You are the world's leading authority!"

I resisted the temptation to disburden their pain this way, quickly, easily. Somehow I had to assure them that their son would receive the best possible medical care without accepting oblation to my ego. They were asking me to play a more creditable imitation of God than the first doctor.

It is another one of those gray days when I must set out for Moriah to meet my newest Sarah and Abraham and Isaac.[39] This new Isaac will survive—I've read that in his medical history—but will the family? If I do not fan the parents' fury, most likely they will find a third brittle point for accord. *Doctors always stick together*, they will say. *What could we have expected?* they will agree. For this and this alone, Jack will take his wife's hand. They will misunderstand my motive when I suggest that they examine their anger if they hope to get rid of the intolerable pain.

In *A Window to Heaven* I wrote of an operatic prologue that echoed a dying child's vision of angels.[40] But it is not those angelic voices that I hear today. Rather, it is the satanic interruption from the same prologue that I recognize in this modern medical scene.

"Vainglorious dust! Overweening atoms!" complains Mephistopheles.[41] The master of evil is bored. Humankind is so debased that there is no one really worth tempting. But then he learns of Faust and Margereta, plots their undoing as man and woman, lovers, parents. Faust sells his soul for youth, Margereta murders their child.

Faust and Margereta, Abraham and Sarah, Cindy and Jack, Dr. Di and their doctor at home—Satan mocks us all. I detect his arrogant intrusion everytime I face Mount Moriah. Two thousand years ago, on another pinnacle, that same sardonic laugh was heard and rebuffed:

> And the devil said to him, "To you I will give their glory and all this authority; for it has been given over to me, and I give it to anyone I please. If you, then, will worship me, it will all be yours." Jesus answered him, "It is written, 'Worship the Lord your God, and serve only him.'"[42]

The first commandment remains simple, to have no other gods before God. Our task on Moriah is to learn what this means in our own families, in our own times, and in our own traditions. On Moriah we are alone with God.

Cindy and Jack are mere mortals. And they, like Abraham, are suffering mortal pain. Moriah's lesson seems perverse, cruel. I ache for the most important human beings in young Ricky's life. It would seem more merciful to extinguish their anguish, accept the offering, their glory and all this authority.

But instead I must admit that I too am a pile of overweening atoms. I must point them away from me if I would offer real healing for their pain. I am reminded of words that were meant for all of us who hurt: "Come unto me, all who labor and are heavy laden, and I will give you rest."[43] These are not the words of a dusty demigod in white. They are an invitation from Christ.

Despite a hell on earth, Cindy and Jack are free to stop their flight. Abraham believed God and it was counted unto him as righteousness. Margereta and Faust repented and Mephistopheles was the loser. In the epilogue, it is the angelic chorus, the sweet sound of redemption, that fills our ears.

$$\approx \quad \approx \quad \approx$$

When Sarah's bone-marrow results are ready, I return to the treatment room with the good news that my little fighter is still in remission. The marrow was chock-full of robust, normal blood cells ready to fight infection, heal her bruises. Not one leukemic cell in sight.

Sarah listens to me, feigning disinterest, sniffing and smiling. Wordlessly, she grants her mother permission to launch preformed tears, heal her mother's pain. Mother dabs both pairs of eyes, echoes both sniff and smile.

I kiss Sarah on the forehead and push my luck a bit. "Now, tell me Sarah. Was that very bad?" I wait patiently, for to answer too quickly would not suit her mood or style.

"No, not really," she allows after an eternity-and-two-halves. Then she redeems me from my pain with a barely audible murmur, a sweet angelic whisper: "I wuv oo."

14

NIAP is Pain Spelled Backward

As a mother comforts her child,
so I will comfort you.

Isaiah 66:13 (NIV)

*D*ear Crumb-bunny,

There's no need for a rooster in the Bone Marrow Unit as long as you are here. When you wake up, everybody rouses! You enjoy starting the day as the center of attention with a team of nurses hoping that you will smile and greet them. The other patients have to wait for their baths.

You've come to love these nurses so much that I can almost believe that you know that Mom and Dad need their rest. "But it's the first time I'll be away from her overnight," Mom said as you were admitted.

"You've been on call in 'solo practice' for a year, Dr. Mom." I try my luck to convince her there are long-term benefits from short-term separation. "It's time for us to carry the beeper and you to get some rest." Fortunately, Mom likes my metaphor.

You are so loved, and none of your lovers has ever paused to question your worthiness. Your pain is not so hard to banish. You are apart from your mom and dad *for a short season and then (in my fantasies) returned to their care until your wedding day.*

I wish it were so for all children.

❧   ❧   ❧

The solution for much pain is not necessarily more medication. Before her bone-marrow transplantation, Crumb-bunny was hospitalized on the regular ward. Visits to that ward remind me that there are other forms of misery, with less hope than cancer, that can visit the young.

A six-week-old in a pram near the nurses' station is crying his heart out with a familiar howl. When I was an intern, we called them "baby junkies." Today they are known in our hospital vernacular as "jit babies," describing their irritable behavior as they withdraw from the narcotics their addict-mothers had abused.

The pain of withdrawal is handled with decreasing doses of narcotic and sedative but an important part of their therapy is never recorded on the chart as such. If the baby becomes too cranky, someone picks it up and holds it in her arms.

I take the infant from his tear-and-sweat-soaked sheet and the crying ceases as he is cradled snuggly, rocked gently. It's hard to rock and write, so my progress notes on charts on that ward have a peculiar jerky quality to the script. I am reminded of Luci Shaw's poem, *Mary's Song:*

Blue homespun and the bend of my breast
keep warm this small hot naked star
fallen to my arms. (Rest . . .
you who have had so far
to come.) Now nearness satisfies
the body of God sweetly.
Quiet he lies, whose vigor
hurled a universe. He sleeps
whose eyelids have not closed before.[44]

The baby's mother has returned to the streets to earn a living, abandoning him to our ward and the state. Some of these babies test positive for HIV as well, like the babe in my arms. He sleeps peacefully and I think of words attributed to Mary's hot naked star: *Whoever welcomes one such child in my name welcomes me.*[45]

It is at times like this I think of my student days and my old chief. I wish he were still alive so that I could share these experiences with him. I recall one of the last times that I saw him before his death. On a day intended to honor him, some of his former students were invited to present scientific papers.

As I gave my medical paper, he beamed approvingly. I scanned the audience, looking for other familiar faces from the past. In the fourth row I spotted another now elderly, retired professor. He was scowling as he listened but I did not think he was disapproving. I was sure he was trying to fix me in time and place, this woman who works only with suffering children.

When science was sated, we adjourned to the faculty dining room for the festivities to continue. Science alone seemed inadequate praise for my old hero so I had composed a song. After lunch I took out my guitar and sang my *Ballad of the Silver Fox*. The chief was delighted. In the crowd I saw another older man, the one who considered pediatrics unsuitable for tenderhearted women. This time, a blaze of recognition transformed his features. He sought me out afterward. "Now I remember you," he said. "You always were a maverick."

The baby stirs in my arms. My paperwork is complete and I have no excuse to linger, so I rock a bit longer while I scan the horizon for another step-in parent to take my place. None is in view so I resume my rocking reverie.

The baby yawns expansively and tries his best to focus on me and the colorful squiggle pinned to my sweater that had brushed against his cheek. This brooch, a cheerful purple worm with blue stripes and a chartreuse bow tie, is my very own NIAP, gift of a teenager who contributed to its unique design.

NIAP is pronounced nāpe. NIAP is pain spelled backwards. As it says in the "owner's manual," every part of the NIAP is very important and has an important purpose. Like the curl on its tail (to help take away pain), the swirl on its body (to help take away boo-boos) and bright, bright colors—just plain nice to see.

The kids who designed it did so in the hope that its presence would assist everyone and anyone in their battle against all pain and hurt. I am one of the privileged few who have a NIAP to color-coordinate with almost any outfit I might wear. Color does not only describe the pain; it can spell out its relief as well.

Can I teach my own students to be the mavericks they were meant to be? An intern spots me with the baby and offers to take the next "shift." As my old chief encouraged me so many years ago to hasten Millie's healing by sharing myself, so I try to encourage the next generation of young doctors.

I kiss the soft sleeping head before passing him on to my maverick-in-training. The sweet perfume of baby shampoo lingers on my sweater as a reminder of how important human companionship is in the relief of pain.

15

Thwarting
the Thief

*The thief comes only to steal and kill
and destroy. I [Jesus] have come
that they might have life, and have
it to the full.*

John 10:10 (NIV).

*D*ear Crumb-bunny,

  My heart sank the day I first met you. The test results weren't back in yet but I knew what the diagnosis was. I've spent too many years stalking that thief. I know his MO all too well and so did your parents.

  Your mother did everything possible to take care of herself and your brother-on-board during her first pregnancy. Except for the mild cold, everything had been perfect. But your brother was born critically ill, and they looked to your mother's history for the answer, wondering whether it was a virus. Mom and Dad laid your brother to rest after an autopsy, hearing that he was carried away by an overwhelming infection, a random piece of poor luck, not a repeatable event.

  At least you were born healthy. But when the fevers began, the terror returned. You came to us, and your parents learned that the autopsy at the other hospital had missed the telltale cells. This was not random bad luck but a disease that kills one out of four of an affected babies' brothers and sisters. The thief was on your trail, seeking to rob you of your life, your parents of their only living child.

We temporized, shutting the thief out with chemotherapy and you revived to win all our hearts. But the thief knows the odds. The predator waits.

We are not satisfied with history repeating itself so we have hidden you away. That old robber cannot find you in our secret kingdom.[46]

❃ ❃ ❃

Each year I see a growing number of families who are poorly prepared for the long journey that lies ahead. There are too many opportunities for isolation available to the "me generation," and the solitary are sitting ducks for the thief.

On one of his old *Prairie Home Companion* radio shows, Garrison Keillor told of an experience at a folk concert. An artist thrilled his audience with a seemingly inspired rendition of Amazing Grace. Keillor felt led to tell the singer how touched he was by the performance and sought him out backstage. To Keillor's disappointment, the vocalist disclaimed that he actually believed any of the words he had just sung. The words had not come from his heart.

To express his disappointment, America's gentle contemporary humorist rewrote the lyrics of John Newton's famous old hymn. He composed an anthem suitable for today, an era that celebrates the self:

Amazing me, how sweet the sound.

Keillor, enriched by grace, refused to let the thief rob him. While "amazing me" suggests introspection and isolation, amazing grace invites connection, reorients from I-I to I-thou and I-Thou.

❦　　❦　　❦

A wealthy man was moving to our area. He visited various cancer centers to determine where his son would receive his further care. The boy still required chemotherapy and careful follow-up. The dad had already checked out each of our doctors. Now he was impressed with our new outpatient area.

This father seemed pleased until we reached the waiting area where a number of young African-American patients happened to be playing that day. The rich man's eyes narrowed and the pitch of his voice changed, "Of course, we will have to work everything around my son's schooling. We will want him to come at the end of the day so that he doesn't miss any classes. I can pay." His body language underlined his words. At the end of the day he hoped that these "other" children would be gone. He never came back.

This rich man let the thief rob him of a priceless treasure. His silver and gold could not buy the riches that we have to offer. There is no price tag on our greatest assets: ourselves and each other. And none of us, black or white, young or old, rich or poor, is less valuable in our family. You can't sneak in by a back door at night after potential "lepers" leave and still gain the best that we have to offer.

In the clinic where families mingle, friendships are solidified, and caring is extended to more than me and mine. There's an occasional solitary figure who slips in and out quickly without exchanging a word or glance with another, but that is the exception. No man, woman, child, or care-bear is an island here.

The mother of a boy with leukemia confided new insight about the communal aspect of the fight. Before her own child was hospitalized, she never knew another sick youngster. Where were they all—in some secret closet? Or was it she who had shut the door to these others and remained in narcissistic darkness until the door was blown open against her will?

This mother is not alone. Many parents of the newly diagnosed ask if there is an epidemic of cancer in their neighborhood. They cannot believe that there always were this many young people with cancer. Until it affected them, they were blind to the extent of illness and suffering that others have already faced.

❧   ❧   ❧

Sarah runs her hand over her own bald head as she clutches her security blanket shyly and approaches a teenager. "Do you have leukemia, too? You don't have any hair." Her nineteen-year-old new friend doesn't have leukemia, but he does have another form of cancer. Tom sits with Alff in his lap. He defies anyone to dare think that he is too old for stuffed stuff.

Tom sits next to his chauffeur-du-jour. This woman, wife of his pastor, clutches a teddy bear. She has an I-dare-you look on her face. By her side is the cane she uses to support herself during flare-ups of severely disabling arthritis. It could serve any shepherdess well, this beautifully carved and ornamented staff that expresses her defiance of the medical mundane. Alff's friend has a fine companion. Childlike but not childish, the pastor's wife is a one-woman crime-prevention unit. She would wonk the thief with her cane if he dared to approach young Tom.

When physicians concentrate only on the technical details of the physical illness, the robbery of grace is abetted. When nurses miss the interactions of body and soul, the loot fills the sack. When the family fails to move from amazing me to amazing grace, the thief emerges victor and moves on to the next victim. The joy of my work is to see how often the family is released from bondage and it is the thief who goes to jail.

16

Getting Airborne

*I still get butterflies. They just fly
in formation.*

Brenda Lee

Dear Crumb-bunny,

You come to your plastic window to greet me with your same sweet smile. You flap your arms by your sides making snow angels in the snow-pure laminar air. I mimic your motion to your delight. If you keep flapping, you'll rise out of your germ-free goldfish bowl!

You settle into your favorite sleeping posture, face turned away as if to shut out all but slumber, diaper-padded bottom raised in salute to the heavens. At this moment, you look very much like a baroque cherub to me. I reach my hand through the protective plastic glove to pat you. You shift slightly in your sleep, saying both "yes" and "no" to my embrace. For now, your dreams are your own.

Sweet dreams, Grandma's little angel.

 governing ❧   ❧   ❧

Why is it that young children like my patients seem to soar in the heavenlies while adults like me flop back down to earth regularly? Or even run. Pastor-author Browne Barr observes that geese fly much faster in formation than one by one.[47] It's tough flying by yourself. High-flying geese need fine-feathered companions. So do mere humans who face the valley of the shadow.

❧   ❧   ❧

In *A Window to Heaven,* I told the story of Naomi. Her dream surrounded her with the love of God in the moment that she knew that her baby would die of cancer.[48] Naomi was so convinced that God's love would manifest itself in a plan for her life that she was content not to know if she would be given the gift of more babies.

It is now eight years since her firstborn died. God's plan has added two more healthy babies to their little family, and the youngest boy, Christian, is now three. At the dinner table he told Naomi, "An angel visited me last night. I liked him, so I invited him to stay the night and come to my birthday party."

It was Christmastime, a season whose symbolism richly recalls angel visitation. Intrigued, his mother enquired, "Did the angel stay the night?"

"No," answered the little one, then added, "He was a baby and he was very sick."

"What did the angel look like?" his astonished mother probed.

"Lots of lights, like a Christmas tree."

Naomi is a wise woman, one who knows when a

three-year-old has closed a topic to further adult inquiry, so she allowed several months to pass before she again brought up Christian's angelic visitor. She asked him what the angel had told him. Christian became very quiet and said, "It's a secret."

I may be an adult, but I'm improving. In the company of these young children and their parents, I am losing my mistrust of things with wings.

What amazes me about my patients is how easily they understand what it means to keep the covenant, to be people of hope. Children who expect to live do not shrink away from those who will likely die. Their parents may find it a lot harder to maintain the closeness with less fortunate families, but they, too, try their best.

Parents of babies with Crumb-bunny's disease have banded together to help each other and help in research. The "FEL fighters" and "FEL angels" belong to the same family. Death does not have the power to separate these parents, to make them fear each other.

Matt had just started his treatment for Burkitt's lymphoma when he met Brian, who is now hospitalized for terminal care. Matt speaks lovingly of the lad, of his prayers for him. He is not afraid to maintain the attachment.

A few short months ago, Brian was hoping that the medicine would cure his cancer, but he did not shrink from visiting Sharon who was close to death. Three months after Sharon's death, her father visits Brian's mom. Brian, who knows that he is now dying, asks Sharon's dad if he has any messages for her in heaven.

The young artist whose paintings grace the jacket covers of my books is herself a recent addition to our hospital family. Not many months ago Korene came through a special form of surgery that removed her cancerous bone and, happily, saved her leg. Although her chances of survival are now 95%, she does not shy away from talking about those who did not survive. For Korene, hope means more than medicine and statistics, so she prays for Brian as well.

In the closing epilogue of *A Window to Heaven*, I acknowledged that I have unanswered questions for God about the death of children. To live with unanswered questions about the death of the very young requires grace to process hope. Baseball legend Dave Dravecky recently reminded me that grace is also needed for survivors.[49] We talked about my young friend Korene, whose tumor is not unlike the one that was removed by amputation, ending his baseball career. Dave thought about Korene and the other brave little players he personally knows. As he talked, his gaze drifted somewhere higher, another plane. He shared some important words of hope that have helped him get airborne:

> But we have this treasure in jars of clay to show that this all-surpassing power is from God and not from us. We are hard-pressed on every side but not crushed; perplexed but not in despair; persecuted but not abandoned; struck down but not destroyed. We always

carry around in our body the death of Jesus, so that the life of Jesus may also be revealed in our body. . . .

Therefore we do not lose heart. Though outwardly we are wasting away, yet inwardly we are being renewed day by day. For our light and momentary troubles are achieving for us an eternal glory that far outweighs them all.

So we fix our eyes not on what is seen, but what is unseen. For what is seen is temporary, but what is unseen is eternal (2 Cor. 4:7–10, 16–18 NIV).

Full of hope, my youngsters and the young-at-heart get airborne. Formation flying is natural for them, these lovers of life, my things with wings. And as hard-pressed, perplexed, crushed, persecuted, and struck down as I sometimes feel when I don't know all the answers, I will not lose heart. With them, I will fix my eyes on that which is eternal yet unseen.

Epilogue:

A Wedding Invitation

Gather the people. Sanctify the congregation; assemble the aged; gather the children, even infants at the breast. Let the bridegroom leave his room, and the bride her canopy.

Joel 2:16 (NRSV)

*D*ear Crumb-bunny,
Today is a life-day that will always be remembered, a landmark medical and personal event. A stranger's marrow is flowing in your veins, introduced by an intravenous tube. Those foreign cells, looking for their new home, spell the difference between your death and your survival. How can anything lifesaving be truly foreign?

How fearfully and wonderfully made you are that these cells know where to go, the way to make both health and history!

You were born to be a history maker. Today will not be the last time. I plan to live long enough to be there on your wedding day. I can just see the headline:

BABY BONE-MARROW RECIPIENT BECOMES A BRIDE.

"Dr. Crumb Bunny was married today at Yale University's Dwight Chapel. The bride wore an ivory silk crêpe moire gown, edged with Victorian lace. The wedding gown was hand-fashioned by her eighty-year-old doctor/grandma.

"The bride graduated with highest honors from Yale Medical School, receiving both M.D. and Ph.D. degrees.

"Dr. Crumb Bunny was awarded the Nobel Prize in Medicine for the identification and cloning of the gene responsible for familial erythrophagocytic lymphohistiocytosis, commonly known as FEL. She is the youngest Yale faculty member ever to receive this prestigious award.

"After a brief honeymoon in Florence, Italy, the couple will attend the International Congress for Gene Therapy for FEL in the same city. The bride will be the keynote speaker at the Congress."

I could fill your whole book with my dreams for you. Dreams are how princesses and grandmas get airborne.

&. &. &.

Most of us chart our lives by mortal-but-sacred events, births, baptisms, bar mitzvahs, graduations, weddings, death—all mark the familial, familiar rites of passage. These events are ancestral recipes, common but by no means mean. Suffused with spices that define their unique place in our families, they cut into our lives on purpose.

My favorite patient happenings are graduations and weddings. Especially weddings. For some patients, I have to wait what seems a lifetime for a meaningful spark of romance to ignite, a good old-fashioned wedding. I suffer through the throes of young love with them and sometimes even assist with their dreams.

ॐ　ॐ　ॐ

A two-year-old came to me from Nigeria, dying of widespread cancer. Chimma's mother would not take her back home without trying any treatment, despite my blunt statistical offering. The child's initial response to the chemotherapy I prescribed was prompt, but there was no reason to believe that she would not die from that tumor within a few brief years. This was no case for standard therapeutic recipes.

Six months later, Chimma was still doing well and I was invited to their cousin's wedding here in Connecticut. Her father sent a traditional Ibo dress and head-wrap for me to wear. At the reception, I was seated at the head table, my role as an honored guest-matriarch defined. I was to supervise the tossing of the bridal bouquet. In this regard, I am something of an expert. I probably hold the world's record for the most bouquets caught. I invited all the little girls to join in and, expert that I am, I knew exactly where the bouquet would land and so arranged my little patient's place in line. After giving the signal for the toss, I stood behind Chimma, guiding the bouquet into her hands. The other guests clucked their approval, sharing my hope that the child could live to be a bride. Her cousin's wedding day, the tossing of her bridal bouquet, were the first events that caused me to ask, "Why not?" Why couldn't Chimma live? Even with her zero statistical chance of survival, Chimma was entitled to hope.

Sometimes it takes symbolic days like wedding days to learn the right questions to ask, to design Books of Hope, and catch Hope Bouquets. In the paradoxical world in which I work, it is painfully easy to love children like Chimma and Crumb-bunny and all the others. You would love them, too, I wager, if you allowed yourself the risk of coming this close, as close as I am, and not worry whether they are guaranteed to survive.

Not long ago author Valerie Bell observed that it is not easy to love other people's children at all, even when they're healthy.[50] It doesn't seem to come naturally to us. I'd like to extend Valerie's thought further, to make us stretch. It is not easy to love other people's adults. It isn't even easy to love your own adults!

Are you willing to stretch enough to love an adult or two that you currently despise, cherishing that company rather than fleeing from their presence? A covenant community wafts up to find other people's children and other people's adults and invite them along on the wing. It may not be easy, it may not even sound possible, but it is part of flying in formation as a people of hope.

＊＊＊ ＊＊＊ ＊＊＊

Chimma caught that bridal bouquet twelve years ago. By all rights, she should be dead, but instead she's a lovely young teenager, smart as a fox. Her father faithfully sends me photos from Nigeria. Her youngest sister is named Diane.

In a few years I will watch my mail, waiting for an wedding invitation, wondering what the airfare is to Lagos that year. Meanwhile, I relish the letters, the photos, the news. All of it is good. In the Ibo tongue, Chimma means just that: "God is good."

＊＊＊ ＊＊＊ ＊＊＊

This notion of wedding imagery to speak of the covenanting community is a biblical one. While I was in medical school, I became disenchanted with all such concepts, what I understood religious thought to be. Ironically, it was my experiences as a doctor at the bedsides of dying children that later led me to reconsider a Christian faith-profession. It was children who were dying who invited me to enter their covenant, to attend a marriage feast.

My youthful experience of Christianity left me so skeptical about most churches that I inclined toward a do-it-yourself, designer-religion. Organized religion seemed highly imperfect to me. I had my own cathedral, acres of virginal woods. I could read the Bible by myself, thank you, and commune with God in private.

But it's hard to read that Book without looking for someone with whom its message can be shared. It's like attending a great performance alone and having no one to jab in the ribs when you get caught up in the ecstasy.

> "Covenant commits more than the individual. God makes his covenant with Abraham, but through that covenant God brings a covenanted community into being that shoulders responsibility as a servant community to others. Otherwise, covenant deteriorates into the commitment of the loner, the physician as solitary gunslinger".[51]

Ironically, at the same time that I was wandering in the woods, I was telling parents of seriously ill children not to be lone gunslingers. I noticed that those parents in my practice who "made it" were those who linked themselves with people of kindred spirit, imperfect as those others might be. Finally, I heard the echo of my own words replayed. I recognized in its echo the discrepancy between my professional advice to parents and my own actions.

This lone gunslinger joined a local family of faith, imperfect as it may be, imperfect as I am. This faith-family has been my sounding board as I continue to seek to integrate my growing faith with my life's work. This is what covenant is all about: uniting with others, extending the invitation, preparing for the feast. It's no fun to dine alone. No bridal party invites only one guest.

The covenanted community is a ravishing bride,

clothed in white fine linen, bright and pure. This is the image that John saw on the isle of Patmos, a gift-vision from a visitor with wings. "Blessed are those who are invited to the marriage supper of the Lamb," the angel said.[52]

Because of the special children who have come into my life, I have set aside many of my presumptions. Things are not at all the way I had supposed. There is reason to hope. Life can defeat death, humor can stand in pathos' place. The weak and foolish lead, and I am often wise enough to follow.

Come, join me, then, dear friend. There's going to be a wedding. But first I must prepare, and so must you if you would come along. Leave your prejudices behind and take off your shoes, here on this holy ground. Don't even think about potential obstacles underfoot. Just lift up your eyes, fix and search for your goal.

You don't need answers to all your weighty questions to come along, only a passion for that which is unseen and eternal. And a heart full of hope. If you seem to lose your way en route to the feast, please don't despair. God knows your every need. He will send a child to lead you.

ॐ   ॐ   ॐ

Hush, little Crumb-bunny. Grandma's here. The bone marrow infusion is now complete. Even though you don't notice, there's a change in you already.

You stand and clap to say hello. But, instead of saluting me with your backwards bye-bye, your tiny hand curves forward to tease me and to greet. Instead of your quaint little wave to yourself, for the first time your palm comes into view. The time has come, little angel, for you to share your secret.

You giggle and prance and show me something new. Finally, the reason for your preoccupation comes into view as you open your pudgy hand to greet me. For the first time I can see your big secret. It is God, unseen yet eternal, who is engraved on the palm on your hand. Come closer, little Sweetie. Come take my hand.

Love, Dr. Di

Afterword

Fourteen days after her bone-marrow transplantation, Crumb-bunny's blood counts started to indicate signs of new life coming from her bone marrow. In record time, her own bone marrow was making normal cells. The gracious gift of life had been accepted. She was now able to defend herself against infection and bleeding. It would not be long before the butterfly could be liberated from her sterile chrysalis.

The Tuesday after Easter, six weeks after her transplant, her mom entered the life island for the first time unmasked, ungloved, ungowned. It was my privilege to be there, on that holy ground.

"Can I kiss her?" she asked. It had been fifty-one days since this young mother was allowed to closely embrace her only living child. "I can actually kiss you!"

She clothed the baby in an Easter frock, bonnet, gloves, and slippers. Even her pacifier was color-coordinated. On her way out the door, Crumb-bunny paused briefly, admired herself in a mirror. She was plainly in awe.

Then the baby toddled out with her parents, not looking back.

THE END

Endnotes

PROLOGUE

1. This is adapted from a story told by Jack Hayford in an address entitled *Shout for Joy;* Boston, January 1992.
2. For more information about familial erythrophagocytic lymphohistiocytosis (FEL) and other forms of histiocytosis you can contact the Histiocytosis Association of America, 609 New York Road, Glassboro, N.J. 08028.

Chapter 1

3. A pediatric oncologist is a specialist in cancer in children. The full title for our speciality is "pediatric hematology-oncology." We also care for children with non-cancerous blood diseases, such as histiocytosis, especially when cancer-type treatments are recommended. For simplicity in this book, I have used the terms "oncology" and "cancer" (which account for 90% of my own patient work) in a broader generic sense than I would in technical writing.
4. Cf. Isaiah 11:6.

Chapter 2

5. The title of a book by Richard Gahman (New York: McGraw-Hill, 1960).

6. *American Heritage Dictionary.*
7. See Chapter 11 of *A Window to Heaven,* 110–11.
8. Matt. 28:20 (NRSV).
9. This pastor's experience is typical. The typical family practitioner, whose patient population is roughly the same size as the typical congregation, will diagnosis cancer in only one child in a long professional career. Neither senior parish clergy nor senior general physicians have extensive personal experience to draw upon when they face that one child.

Chapter 3

10. Within the last few months I have heard multiple variations on this story, all of which are probably retelling of the same original story. Since all of these reports were secondhand or later, I am hesitant to cite any one as the "correct" version. If the children's parents happen to read this note, I would be delighted to hear from them so that the accurate details and proper credit can be given. Until then, I will treat the story as a delightful allegory.
11. Jackie Pullinger with Andrew Quick, *Chasing the Dragon* (London: Hodder and Stoughton, 1980), 224–25.

Chapter 4

12. "Grand Rounds" is the major teaching conference of each week in most medical school departments.

Chapter 5

13. Paul S. Minear, *Eyes of Faith* (Philadelphia: Westminster Press, 1956), 14.
14. Leanne Payne, *The Healing Presence* (Wheaton: Crossways, 1989), 23.

Chapter 6

15. Professor Paul Ramsey quotes here theologian Karl Barth in Ramsey, Paul, *The Patient As a Person: Explorations in Medical Ethics* (New Haven: Yale University Press, 1970).

16. William F. May, *A Physician's Covenant: Images of the Healer in Medical Ethics* (Philadelphia: Westminster Press, 1983).

17. Peschel, Richard E. and Enid Rhodes Peschel: *When a Doctor Hates a Patient and Other Chapters in a Young Physician's Life* (Berkeley: University of California Press, 1986), 118.

18. Siegel, Bernie: *Love, Medicine and Miracles* (New York: Harper & Row, 1986), 220.

19. Matt. 25:29 (NRSV).

Chapter 8

20. Matt. 21:16 (NRSV).

21. "Dartmouth Redesigns Medical Training to Give Future Doctors a Human Touch," *New York Times* (September 2, 1992), B 7.

Chapter 9

22. Morris West uses the term, "Les petite bouffonnes du bon Dieu" for Down's syndrome in his wonderful novel, *The Clowns of God* (New York: William Morrow & Co., 1981).

23. Apple Doll House was a project of S.A.R.A.H. (Shoreline Association for the Retarded and Handicapped), Guilford, Ct.

24. "The poignant thoughts of Down's children are given voice," *New York Times* (December 22, 1987), C 1, 9.

25. Harold H. Wilke, *Creating the Caring Congregation* (Nashville: Abington, 1980), foreword. Dr. Wilke is director of The Healing Community, 138 Alsworth Avenue, N.Y. 10606.

26. Cf. Lev. 21:18–21 (NRSV).

Chapter 10

27. (San Francisco: Harper & Row, 1979), xv.

28. John 14:27 (NRSV).

29. Elisabeth Kübler-Ross, *On Death and Dying* (New York: Macmillan Company, 1969).

30. Shiela Cassidy, *Sharing the Darkness* (London: Darton, Longman & Todd, 1988), 3. Cf. Luke 4:11–18.

31. Conrad Hyers, "Easter Hilarity," in *And God Created Laughter: The Bible As Divine Comedy* (Atlanta: John Knox Press, 1987), 24–28. (Quoted by Doris Donnelly in *Divine Folly: Being Religious and the Exercise of Humor, Theology Today,* January 1992, 385–98).

32. 1 Cor. 15:54, 55 (NRSV).

Chapter 11

33. John 9:2, 3 (NIV).

34. John 9:3 (NIV).

Chapter 12

35. Matt. 10:39 (NRSV).

36. Paraphrased by J. B. Phillips in *Your God Is Too Small* (New York: Macmillan, 1964), 120.

Chapter 13

37. Prov. 3:5, 6 (NRSV)

38. In his book *A Road Less Traveled* (New York: Simon & Schuster, 1978), psychiatrist M. Scott Peck warns that

the tendency to avoid pain is "the primary basis of all mental illness."

39. From "Facing Mount Moriah" in *A Window to Heaven*.
40. From "A Choir of Angels" in *A Window to Heaven*.
41. Translation of the Mephistopheles libretto by DECCA 1984 Avril Bardoni.
42. Luke 4:6–8 (NRSV)
43. Matt. 11:28

Chapter 14

44. Luci Shaw and Timothy R. Botts, *Horizon-Exploring Creation* (Grand Rapids: Zondervan, 1992), 114.
45. Matt. 18:5 (NRSV).
46. I am indebted to Kyle and Leslie Pruett for introducing me to the notion of serious illness as a thief.
47. Browne Barr, *High-Flying Geese: Unexpected Reflections on the Church and Its Ministry* (New York: Seabury Press, 1983), 19.
48. Cf. "Learning a New Language," 74–77.
49. Dave Dravecky tells his story in two books: *Comeback* (Grand Rapids: Zondervan, 1990) and *When You Can't Come Back* (Grand Rapids: Zondervan, 1992).

Epilogue

50. Valerie Bell is the author of a book entitled, *Nobody's Children* (Dallas: Word Books, 1989).
51. From *The Physician's Covenant*.
52. Rev. 19:9 (NRSV).